Management of Menopause

Management of Menopause

Shaikh Zinnat Ara Nasreen
MBBS MPH FCPS MRCOG FRCOG FIAOG
Professor and Head
Department of Obstetrics and Gynecology
ZH Sikder Women's Medical College and Hospital
Dhaka, Bangladesh

Forewords
Shahla Khatun
TA Chowdhury

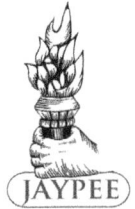

JAYPEE BROTHERS MEDICAL PUBLISHERS
The Health Sciences Publisher
New Delhi | London

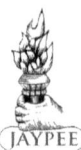 **Jaypee Brothers Medical Publishers (P) Ltd**

Headquarters

Jaypee Brothers Medical Publishers (P) Ltd
EMCA House, 23/23-B
Ansari Road, Daryaganj
New Delhi 110 002, India
Landline: +91-11-23272143, +91-11-23272703
+91-11-23282021, +91-11-23245672
Email: jaypee@jaypeebrothers.com

Corporate Office

Jaypee Brothers Medical Publishers (P) Ltd
4838/24, Ansari Road, Daryaganj
New Delhi 110 002, India
Phone: +91-11-43574357
Fax: +91-11-43574314
Email: jaypee@jaypeebrothers.com

Overseas Office

JP Medical Ltd
83 Victoria Street, London
SW1H 0HW (UK)
Phone: +44 20 3170 8910
Fax: +44 (0)20 3008 6180
Email: info@jpmedpub.com

Website: www.jaypeebrothers.com
Website: www.jaypeedigital.com

© 2022, Jaypee Brothers Medical Publishers

The views and opinions expressed in this book are solely those of the original contributor(s)/author(s) and do not necessarily represent those of editor(s) of the book.

All rights reserved. No part of this publication may be reproduced, stored or transmitted in any form or by any means, electronic, mechanical, photocopying, recording or otherwise, without the prior permission in writing of the publishers.

All brand names and product names used in this book are trade names, service marks, trademarks or registered trademarks of their respective owners. The publisher is not associated with any product or vendor mentioned in this book.

Medical knowledge and practice change constantly. This book is designed to provide accurate, authoritative information about the subject matter in question. However, readers are advised to check the most current information available on procedures included and check information from the manufacturer of each product to be administered, to verify the recommended dose, formula, method and duration of administration, adverse effects and contraindications. It is the responsibility of the practitioner to take all appropriate safety precautions. Neither the publisher nor the author(s)/editor(s) assume any liability for any injury and/or damage to persons or property arising from or related to use of material in this book.

This book is sold on the understanding that the publisher is not engaged in providing professional medical services. If such advice or services are required, the services of a competent medical professional should be sought.

Every effort has been made where necessary to contact holders of copyright to obtain permission to reproduce copyright material. If any have been inadvertently overlooked, the publisher will be pleased to make the necessary arrangements at the first opportunity. The **CD/DVD-ROM** (if any) provided in the sealed envelope with this book is complimentary and free of cost. **Not meant for sale.**

Inquiries for bulk sales may be solicited at: jaypee@jaypeebrothers.com

Management of Menopause

First Edition: **2022**

ISBN: 978-93-90595-88-4

Dedicated to

My parents, My husband
My children, My siblings
All the women of Bangladesh

Contributors

Laila Arjumand Banu MBBS FCPS
Senior Consultant
Department of Obstetrics and
Gynecology
LABAID Specialized Hospital
Dhaka, Bangladesh
Past President
Obstetrical and Gynaecological Society
of Bangladesh (OGSB)

Latifa Shamsuddin MBBS FCPS FCPS
(Pak) FICS (USA)
Former Chairperson and Head
Department of Obstetrics and
Gynecology
Bangabandhu Sheikh Mujib Medical
University Hospital
Dhaka, Bangladesh

Md Samiul Huq
MBBS MPH DDSc (UK) MSc (UK) Dermatology
Former Senior Consultant
Department of Dermatology
Square Hospital
Dhaka, Bangladesh

Rowshan Ara Begum MBBS FCPS
Former Head
Department of Obstetrics and Gynecology
Holy Family Red Crescent Medical
College and Hospital
Dhaka, Bangladesh
Past President
Obstetrical and Gynaecological Society
of Bangladesh (OGSB)

Sameena Chowdhury MBBS FCPS
Former Head
Institute of Child and Mother Health
Dhaka, Bangladesh
President
Obstetrical and Gynaecological Society
of Bangladesh (OGSB)

Shaikh Zinnat Ara Nasreen
MBBS MPH FCPS MRCOG FRCOG FIAOG
Professor and Head
Department of Obstetrics and Gynecology
ZH Sikder Women's Medical College and
Hospital
Dhaka, Bangladesh

Suraiya Rahman Brig Gen
Former Advisor Specialist Head
Department of Obstetrics and Gynecology
Combined Military Hospital
Dhaka, Bangladesh

Foreword

It is my great pleasure to write a foreword for *Management of Menopause* by Professor Shaikh Zinnat Ara Nasreen and her contributors. The menopause age is not changed but the women's life expectancy has prolonged (73.3 years in Bangladesh), so women have to live long with menopause and its consequences particularly osteoporosis and cardiovascular diseases.

In 1990, there were 467 million women aged 50 years or more; worldwide, they will number 1,200 million in 2030. The increasing proportion of the aged in the population is posing significant new challenges to politics, society and medicine as well. There is need for comprehensive holistic approach for these women's health and menopause to improve their quality-of-life.

I have gone through the book several times, I found, this book addressed the relationship of biophysiological changes and estrogens deficiency elaborately. Also it provides evidence-based information about the healthy lifestyle, which is the cornerstone of menopause management. The Menopause Hormone Therapy is the topic of controversy since the result of Women's Health Initiative. But this book tried to cover the safety, efficacy, risks, benefits, doses, and route of Menopause Hormone Therapy in the light of latest research. I felt this book will up-to-date and build the capacity of gynecologists and other colleagues in the management of menopause health. The book is written in simple language with lots of references that may prove more interesting and effective way of learning. The book highlighted the management of mental health, skin care and postmenopausal bleeding along with vasomotor symptoms, bone health, cardiovascular health, and genitourinary syndrome of menopause.

I wish that author's evidence-based information will promote the practical application of the contents for improving the quality life of our menopause women.

Writing this foreword has been a very pleasurable and educational experience for me. I have deep appreciation to the author for providing me with this memorable opportunity.

Shahla Khatun
MBBS FRCOG (London) FCPS FICS
National Professor
President
Bangladesh Menopause Society

Foreword

It gives me great pleasure to write a few words about the unique monograph on menopause written by Prof Shaikh Zinnat Ara Nasreen, currently working as Professor of Obstetrics and Gynecology at ZH Sikder Women's Medical College and Hospital, Dhaka, Bangladesh.

Menopause is a unique period in a woman's life cycle. Proper management of menopause not only improves the quality-of-life but can also prevent long-term suffering and disability. Even half-a-century ago women lived for a short period after, and the need for management during this short period was not considered to be a priority. Many women considered the menopausal symptoms as the normal price to pay for ageing and often did not consult a physician for the relief of symptoms.

Situation has changed dramatically now. Women are living longer in both developed and developing countries and spend at least one-third of their life span in menopause. Menopause can cause many pathophysiological changes, both physical and psychological. Proper understanding of these changes and appropriate intervention can greatly improve the quality-of-life. Menopause also provides opportunity for taking many preventable measures, which can prevent long-term disability.

Many of our doctors who deals with aged women do not have the appropriate knowledge regarding the problems of menopause, and women do not get appropriate and rational treatment. Many of them also suffer from different type of psychological problems and need sympathetic attention from her physician for amelioration of her symptoms.

Prof Shaikh Zinnat Ara Nasreen has tried to discuss different aspects of menopause in different chapters and has tried to give the appropriate solutions without talking too much about the basics and research findings.

I presume that this book has been written aiming to doctors who deal with elderly women such as general practitioners and gynecologists, who will find this book to be very useful in their clinical practice.

It will also be reference volume for others who wants to know about menopause and its implication for women's health.

To my knowledge not many books on rational, scientific and up-to-date management of menopause is available currently in this country and this book will fill up the void.

I have every hope this book will be very well-accepted by its readers.

TA Chowdhury (Shadhinota Podok Awardee)
FRCS FFRCOG FCPS RCP PhD
Honorary Professor of Obstetrics and Gynecology
Ibrahim Medical College and BIRDEM
Dhaka, Bangladesh

Preface

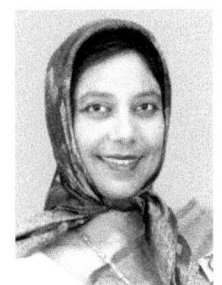

Since life expectancy has increased, a woman spends approximately more than one-third of her life in the postmenopausal period, hence, providing high quality welfare and health care for menopause women is of great importance in order to prevent long-term complications, particularly *cardiovascular disorder and osteoporosis*. In 1990, there was 467 million women aged 50 years, and by 2030, this global figure is expected to 1,200 million (according to World Health Organization). This demographic and epidemiological shift would result in the non-communicable diseases to be the major cause of morbidity in the middle age and older women. However, being most notable event of midlife, the menopause is overlooked. So better understanding of menopause, its consequences and management are the topmost priority. A well-managed menopause transition sets the stage of active and healthy aging. The genesis of this book is to arm the reader with practical knowledge in how to recognize, address, and treat (preventive and curative) optimally the most modern-time menopause issues and its consequences.

From last three decades, menopause is gaining much better understanding. Across the world, constant publication of clinical trials and other researches are posing challenges to get the nutshell. There are lot of debates and controversies about the treatment particularly the use of menopause hormone therapy. Thus, for practitioners, it is becoming increasingly difficult to be able to form a well-balanced view about, menopause care and menopause hormone therapy. This book will provide evidence-based framework for practitioners to manage menopause with the holistic approach including the lifestyle modification and menopause hormone therapy, if indicated, to improve the quality-of-life of women.

I felt the overwhelming demand of updated knowledge on "menopause care" among our gynecologists and other colleagues. Therefore, this book will try to provide comprehensive cutting-edge information regarding menopause health. With this book, physicians, gynecologists, residents and postgraduate students will confidently acquire updated knowledge about menopause care and be able to practically apply their knowledge toward real-world clinical settings. Its value is further enhanced by having plenty references material for the clarification.

I acknowledge the contributors and the reviewers for their kind efforts to enrich this book.

I would like to pay my respect and gratitude to all my well-wishers whose continuous support encouraged and inspired me to prepare this book.

I sincerely hope this comprehensive book will be useful to update and enable the menopause care providers to give optimal preventive and curative treatment to improve the quality-of-life for women with menopause and beyond.

Shaikh Zinnat Ara Nasreen

Acknowledgments

My heartfelt thanks to all who, contributed in this book. I acknowledge, with deep gratitude, national Professor Shahla Khatun for her continuous support and writing the foreword for me. I am extremely honored and would like to express my heartfelt gratefulness and respect to Prof TA Chowdhury for giving a valuable comment for my book. Also I am grateful to all my teachers. I must acknowledge my colleagues and well-wishers for their gracious support and encouragement.

Contents

1. Introduction to Menopause — 1
2. How to Diagnose Menopause? — 14
3. Nutrition, Exercise and Lifestyle for Menopause Women — 21
4. Vasomotor Symptoms and Menopause — 30
5. Genitourinary Syndrome of Menopause — 44
6. Osteoporosis, Bone Health, and Menopause — 61
7. Cardiovascular Health and Menopause — 81
8. Brain, Cognition and Menopause — 92
9. Sexuality and Menopause — 103
10. Contraceptives in Perimenopause — 110
11. Skin Care and Menopause — 119
12. Mental Health and Menopause — 131
13. Premature Ovarian Insufficiency — 140
14. Metabolic Syndrome and Menopause — 156
15. Postmenopausal Bleeding — 168
16. Risk and Benefits of Menopausal Hormone Therapy — 180
17. Prescribing Hormone Replacement Therapy — 190

Index — *209*

CHAPTER 1
Introduction to Menopause

■ INTRODUCTION

Menopause is a normal physiological and natural event of women's life. Menopause is a transition into a new phase of life. It begins when the menstrual cycle finishes forever. It is an inevitable component of aging and encompasses the loss of ovarian reproductive function, either occurring spontaneously or secondary to other conditions. Menopause is the permanent cessation of menstruation in a non-hysterectomized woman. As a woman with an intact uterus may have stopped menstruating for a range of reasons, such as having had an endometrial ablation or a hormonal intrauterine device (IUD) inserted, a more pragmatic approach is to define menopause as the permanent cessation of ovarian function.

The decline in ovarian estrogen production at menopause can cause physical symptoms that may be debilitating, including hot flushes night sweats, urogenital atrophy, sexual dysfunction, mood changes, bone loss, and metabolic changes that predispose to cardiovascular disease and diabetes. Age of menopause is not being changed since ancient period but life expectancy of women is prolonged over the years, therefore women has to spent more than one-third of their lifespan in menopause with the consequences.

The age of menopause somehow environmental and genetically determined, this means that mothers and daughters experience menopause at about the same age. There is also some evidence to suggest that women reach menopause earlier if they have a lot of children or smoke a lot. Being underweight or overweight and the length of a woman's menstrual cycle can also influence when her menopause starts. During the transition to menopause and beyond, the hormone estrogen begins to decline because ovaries stop producing steroid hormone.

In postmenopause, declining estrogen levels are associated with the consequences of menopause include:
- Vasomotor events (hot flushes)
- Insomnia
- Weight gain
- Mood changes
- Irregular menses
- Breast pain
- Depression, and discomfort associated with genitourinary atrophy and vaginal dryness.[1-6]

Although the onset may vary, natural menopause typically occurs between the ages of 45 and 55 years and is regarded as a midlife event.

The exact age of menopause may be influenced by several factors, including the following:
- Geographical location
- Race/ethnicity
- Body mass index (BMI) or body composition
- Physical activity, diet
- Smoking and parity.

Factors that associated with a younger age at menopause include:
- Living at high altitudes
- Malnourishment
- Low socioeconomic status
- Cigarette smoking.

Conversely, factors that are associated with older age at menopause include:
- Taller height
- Heavier bodyweight
- Higher number of childbirths
- Alcohol consumption
- Oral contraceptive use.

Though natural events of estrogen deficiency of menopause herald a variety of potential problems that can affect the quality-of-life, specific concerns include subjective symptoms such as vasomotor instability, psychosocial, cognitive disorders, genitourinary dysfunction, metabolic changes, and osteoporosis. The individual' experience of the menopause transition varies widely, many women may suffer from depression, anxiety, and low mood during menopause. It is not unusual to experience times of irritability and crying spells.

Different women may experience this phase of their life very differently. Around menopause, various physical and mental changes can occur, causing symptoms. Some of these start before menopause and some continue after it.

Only few have severe menopause-related problems over a long period of time. Important influential factors include the age at which menopause occurs, personal health well-being, and each woman's environment and culture. Menopause can also have some positive effects, although they often go unmentioned. It makes contraception and menstrual problems a thing of the past. If a woman used to have heavy, painful periods or endometriosis, her quality-of-life might actually improve a lot. Migraines sometimes go away after menopause. For generation, women have dealt with dynamic changes in their body and mind. In our society, menopausal symptoms are regarded as normal symptom of transition and will fade with years and aging but unfortunately issues evolve of weak bones, susceptibility to cancer, endocrine, metabolic cardiovascular disorders, and psychiatric illness which remain unaddressed. Nevertheless in this modern arena, women should not suffer silently, that need to be addressed to improve the quality of their lives.

Therefore gynecologists, doctors have to refine their skill for menopause management with better information of lifestyle modification, hormone therapy, nonhormone medications, sexual dysfunction, urogenital discomfort, and most importantly the enormous benefits of exercise and right approach to nutrition and diet. Both healthcare providers and the postmenopause women deserve an understanding of the basis of menopause and basis for therapeutic recommendation aimed at relieving symptoms, improving quality-of-life and reducing the subsequent health risks.

▪ DEFINITION

Natural menopause is recognized to have occurred after 12 consecutive months of amenorrhea, for which there is no other obvious pathological or physiological cause. Menopause occurs with the final menstrual period (FMP), which is known with certainty only in retrospect a year or more after the event. An adequate independent biological marker for the event does not exist. If a woman would like to be surer about whether she has entered the menopause, her blood sample can be measured for follicle-stimulating hormone (FSH) level. But checking hormone levels has little practical value, unless somebody is having premature menopause.

Perimenopause is the transitional time that starts couple of years before menopause and includes the 12 months that follow a person's last period. It occurs on average at age 47 years.[7]

During perimenopause, i.e., immediately prior to the menopause, the endocrinological, biological, and clinical features approaches towards menopause. As ovaries gradually produce less and less hormones, and fewer eggs during perimenopause, woman may develop irregular cycles of anovulation and menstruation leading up to menopause and continuing until 12 months after her final period.

Menopause is reached when the last egg is released and 1 year passed from the last date of menstruation.

Menopausal transition: The term "menopausal transition" should be reserved for the time before the FMP when variability in the menstrual cycle is usually increased. This term can be used synonymously with "pre-menopause".

Menopause starts either 12 months after the last period or when menstruation has stopped or for the removal of the ovaries for clinical reason.

Postmenopause refers to the years after menopause, although it can be difficult to know when menopause finished and postmenopause starts.

TABLE 1: STRAW SYSTEM (Stages of Reproductive Ageing Workshop).

Stages	−5	−4	−3	−2	−1		+1	+2
Terminology	Reproductive			Menopausal transition			Postmenopause	
	Early	Peak	Late	Early	Late		Early	Late
				Perimenopause				
Duration of stage	Variable			Variable		1 year	4 years	Until demise
Menstrual cycles	Variable to regular	Regular		Variable cycle length (>7 days different from normal)	>2 skipped cycles and an interval of amenorrhea	12 months amenorrhea	None	
Endocrine	Normal FSH		↑ FSH	↑ FSH			↑ FSH	

Source: Soules MR, Sherman S, Parrott E, Rebar R, Santoro N, Utian W, et al. Executive summary: Stages of Reproductive Aging Workshop (STRAW). Fertil Steril. 2001;76:874-8.

Relationship between different time periods surrounding the menopause (modified from WHO 96238) is described in **Table 1**.

■ CONSEQUENCES OF MENOPAUSE

Menstrual Irregularities

Menstrual irregularities are a common complaint during menopause transition. Infrequent ovulation and anovulation lead to changes in the length of proliferative phase, and in the absence of progesterone, decline of estrogen lead to heavier and irregular menstruation.[8] In some women scanty periods with long cycles may be the main symptom. The first sign that menopause is approaching is usually periods occurring less regularly. They may come more or less frequently than usual, and they may be heavier or lighter.

However, postcoital bleeding, prolonged bleeding, and postmenopausal bleeding require further investigation to rule out any hidden malignancy.

Vasomotor Symptoms

Vasomotor symptoms are the main bothering symptoms in the early menopause. They include hot flushes, night sweats, and are termed vasomotor symptoms because of vascular reactivity with initial prominent vasodilation. Hot flushes are transient periods of intense heat in the upper part of the body usually accompanied by sweating. Its exact mechanism is not known, but is believed to be due to narrowing of thermoregulatory zone of hypothalamus with decline of estrogen level. Hot flushes and night sweats are experienced by about 50–80% of menopausal women,[9-11] which is mild form and in about 20-25%, it can be severe to cause significant distress, for which women may seek advice.[12,13] Sleep disturbances caused by hot flushes and sweating can lead to lethargy, poor physical functioning, and depressed mood. In about 25% of women, hot flushes may continue for over 5 years; in a small percentage of women, it may continue up to 10 years or more. Some people experience night sweats and cold flushes, or chills, in addition to or instead of hot flushes. In surgical menopause, vasomotor symptoms are abrupt and severe. Low body weight, lack of exercise, and smoking are risk factors for hot flushes.

Severity, frequency and duration of hot flushes vary with menopausal status, ethnicity, age, cultural factors, and woman's perception of menopause. In many western countries and Australia, 60-80% of women experience hot flushes, while the prevalence is 20-30% in the Chinese and Japanese women. In Asia, 40-60% of women have hot flushes. Recent studies indicate an association of hot flushes with morbid conditions such as cardiovascular disease, osteoporosis, fragility fractures, and diabetes.[9]

Mood Disorders

Mood swing, anxiety, and depression are some of the psychological symptoms during menopausal change. Nearly half of women on menopause transition can get easily irritated. They become less patient with the members of the family, friends, and colleagues and often feel tired and sad. With emotional changes, they can appear nervous, stressful, and sometimes aggressive. Mood swings are due to changes in serotonin activity following estrogen decline but may also be caused by other menopausal symptoms as hot flushes and night sweats.

Anxiety in the form of nervousness, worries, or panic attacks may occur during perimenopause. Hormonal changes, vasomotor symptoms, and midlife stresses contribute to anxiety during this period. Panic disorders are associated with negative life events, impairment of activity, or physical illnesses. In peri- or postmenopausal women who report sleep disturbances, treating the vasomotor symptoms may decrease sleep disturbances, but this may not resolve all sleep problems, as there are many other things that can disturb sleep, such as primary sleep disorders, anxiety, and depression.[14]

Depression is more common in the menopause transition. Those who had previous episodes of depression are at a higher risk. Depression is associated with hormonal changes during this period, stressful life events, poor sleep, hot flushes, employment status, ethnicity, and cultural attitudes. While feelings of sadness, irritability, and tiredness are common during menopause, they do not necessarily indicate depression unless it persists for longer period.

Insomnia may be seen in some women and they are more likely to have anxiety, stress, and depressive disorders. Sleep disorders are associated with menopause transition and influenced by presence of hot flushes, psychosocial problems, and by some medication. Sleep apnea too may occur during this period, and obese women are at a higher risk.

Genitourinary Symptoms

Estrogen receptors are present abundantly in the vagina, vestibule, and trigone area of the bladder. With estrogen deficiency after menopause, many anatomical and physiological changes occur in this area. With reduced collagen and hyaline content and thinning of vaginal epithelium labia minora appear thin and atrophic leading to dyspareunia. Higher predisposition to vaginal infection is attributed to rise in vaginal pH due to loss of vaginal glycogen. Dryness, loss of elasticity, and flexibility of vagina contribute to epithelial damage, and irritation and bleeding after intercourse. On examination, the vagina seems short and narrow, with the absence of rugae and appears pale. Symptoms of vaginal atrophy along with urinary symptoms are collectively designated as genitourinary syndrome of menopause (GSM).

Along with dyspareunia, repeated urinary tract infection (UTI), nocturia, urge incontinence, and stress incontinence are the common urinary symptoms in the postmenopausal age. About 20–30% of postmenopausal women have urgency and have urinary incontinence. With genital prolapse, women may suffer from recurrent UTIs.

Sexual Function

Estrogen deficiency leads to a decrease in blood flow to the vagina and vulva. This decrease is a major cause of decreased vaginal lubrication and sexual dysfunction in menopausal women.[15]

Osteoporosis

Accelerated osteoclastic activity, reduced osteoblastic activity, and calcitonin activity due to reduced estrogen and aging process lead to osteoporosis. The incidence of fractures increases, particularly of distal radius, vertebral body, and upper femur. Wedge compression fractures of the spine lead to backache. Bone loss is accelerated soon after menopause. Osteoporosis-related fractures of the hip, vertebra, and pelvis are a common cause of morbidity and mortality in postmenopause women. At the beginning all women should adopt the strategies to prevent osteoporosis and fracture. Women must follow adequate calcium and vitamin D intake, participating in weight-bearing exercise, and avoiding tobacco and excess alcohol consumption. Women should be screened for osteoporosis who are having fragility fracture. If diagnosis is made, they should be offered pharmacologic therapy. Choice of therapy should be based on safety, cost, convenience, and other patient-related factors. Bisphosphonates are often first-line therapy based on efficacy, safety, and cost. Menopause hormone therapy (MHT) has role to prevent bone loss. Osteoporosis is estimated to affect 200 million women worldwide. Awareness regarding osteoporosis is very important at the time of menopause transition.

Cardiovascular Disease

With the loss of cardioprotective action of estrogen by its action on lipids, endothelial function, and anti-inflammatory effect, menopausal women are more liable to get cardiovascular disease. Symptoms of coronary heart disease (CHD) in women are somewhat different from typical male type of angina, which are usually brought by exertion and relieved by rest. Women with myocardial infarction have atypical symptoms such as fatigue, shortness of breath, and atypical chest pain. Many may have nonobstructive coronary heart disease angiogram may not show typical obstruction in the coronary arteries. CHD is the most common cause of death among postmenopausal women; the ratio of CHD in men and women becomes 1:1 after menopause. Women having risk factors or symptoms need full evaluation of cardiovascular diseases. Though high-density lipoprotein (HDL) does not decreased but study suggested that the protective effect of HDL may decrease as women transition to menopause.[16]

Obesity

Menopause itself is not associated with an increased risk of obesity but a shift to an abdominal fat distribution with associated increase visceral adiposity, decreased calorie requirement, more sedentary work after menopause may lead to weight gain. Gynecoid shape (pear shaped) of women may changes to android shape (apple shaped). Abdominal adiposity in body composition at menopause may be caused by the decrease in circulating estrogen. For fat distribution shifts, the relative increase in the androgen-estrogen ratio is likely to be important. Large majority of these women have an increased BMI and waist circumference. Midsection fat distribution is pronounced during menopause and afterwards, and is associated with more risk of development of cardiovascular diseases and metabolic syndrome.

Skin Changes

Dry skin and wrinkling are due to the loss of subcutaneous fat and changes in composition of connective tissue. Dry hair and hair loss, and increased facial hair are caused by reduction in estrogen and relative increase in male hormones. Skin becomes less elastic and wrinkling appears. Nails become brittle and nail growth becomes slow.

Joints

Osteoarthritis is more common in females after menopause, and many epidemiological and clinical studies indicate estrogen deficiency as one of the etiological factors in addition to familial tendency, obesity, and aging. In menopausal women, the knees and hands are mostly affected. While women who are obese or depressed are more likely to experience joint pain, and there also appears to be an association with menopausal status, with peri- and postmenopausal women experiencing more joint pain than premenopausal women.[17]

Sarcopenia

Menopausal transition is associated with accelerated loss of fat-free mass and muscle mass. Decline in resting metabolic rate, decreased activities, and more sedentary habits of postmenopause women results increased central body fatness. Sarcopenia is caused by complex factors but aging and loss of muscle mass due to hormonal changes at menopause. Low levels of physical activity, reduced protein intake and increased oxidative stress are the other compound factors.

Eyes

Postmenopausal women are at a higher risk of developing age-related macular degeneration and association with estrogen deficiency has been suggested. Dry eye syndrome is common in menopause women.

Teeth

In menopausal woman, osteoporosis may lead to loss of the alveolar bone of the jaws, resulting in periodontal disease, loose teeth, and tooth loss. Estrogen therapy has been shown to increase the alveolar bone mass.

Memory Loss

As estrogen has positive effect on cognitive function and neurotransmitters, slight memory loss has been noted at menopause, especially episodic memory and verbal fluency. Estrogen therapy at menopause, whether reduce the risk of dementia and mild cognitive impairment is a matter of debate.

Alzheimer's Disease

Alzheimer's disease is more common in postmenopausal women than in men of same age. It is accompanied by progressive cognitive impairment and reduces the quality-of-life of the woman. These women have memory loss, confusion, and are unable to recognize family members and friends. Often they have repetitive statements and movements, and may have difficulty in getting up from a chair. But whether this is due to menopause is still a matter of controversy.

■ PHYSIOLOGY OF MENOPAUSE

The oocytes in the ovaries undergo atresia throughout a woman's life, and the follicles decline markedly in the mid-thirties. The aging follicles become more resistant to gonadotropin stimulating and circulating FSH and luteinizing hormone (LH). So FSH level increases after menopause. With the loss of functioning ovarian follicles there is a significant decrease in circulating estrogen levels. Inhibin A and B levels also drop at this time due to negative feedback of increased FSH levels. Androstenedione from postmenopausal ovarian theca cell and adrenals is aromatized to estrogen in the granulosa cell and peripheral adipose tissue. There is a small but significant fall of testosterone, androstenedione and sex hormone-binding globulin (SHBG) with menopause. Plasma level of anti-Müllerian hormone (AMH), which correlates with the ovarian reserve, becomes undetectable at menopause.

Premature Menopause

Premature menopause refers to menopause that occurs before the age of 40 years. Also premature menopause occurs with bilateral oophorectomy, following chemotherapy or radiotherapy, or in primary ovarian failure commonly due to immune mechanisms. It occurs in about 1% of women who have abrupt and severe menopausal symptoms and early complications, requiring definitive treatment. They are at high risk of osteoporosis and cardiovascular diseases. These women may need discussion about MHT.

Menopausal symptoms such as hot flushes, mood changes, genitourinary atrophy, sexual dysfunction, etc., may begin in the perimenopause and extend to early and late menopause. They can be severe enough to affect quality-of-life. With the loss of cardioprotective effect of natural estrogen, postmenopausal women are more prone to develop coronary heart disease. Bone mineral density markedly falls and women are more likely to have osteoporosis and resultant fragility fractures, which is a major socioeconomic problem. In addition, metabolic syndrome and gynecological cancers contribute to noncommunicable diseases. Aging and estrogen deficiency may result in degenerative conditions, and deposition of beta amyloid in the brain, which is associated with Alzheimer's disease.

Physiological Changes

Menopause occurs when the ovaries run out of eggs. The basic reproductive unit of the ovary is the ovarian follicle. Each ovarian follicle contains a single oocyte. A female infant at birth has approximately 300,000 ovarian follicles. By approximately 37 years of age, this number is depleted to about 25,000, and at menopause few/none remain.

Loss of ovarian follicles is associated with diminished estradiol (E2) and ovarian inhibin production, and increased production of pituitary FSH. Loss of follicles also results in a fall in the production of AMH which is actually produced by developing ovarian follicles. When follicle numbers decline, AMH levels fall. Hence, AMH levels decline with age. Measurement of AMH is useful in predicting ovarian response to ovulation induction (low level predicts a poor response). But for routine diagnosis and management of menopause, AMH estimation is not required.

Changes in FSH, E2, inhibin B and AMH may precede or coincide with the development of menstrual irregularity or symptoms. After menopause, FSH level become very high, i.e., > 25 mL/L. Again routinely it is not measured but for premature ovarian insufficiency (POI), FSH is measured twice at an interval of 4 months to diagnosis POI.

The stages of menopause have been classified by the Stages of Reproductive Aging Workshop (STRAW), most recently updated as STRAW + 10 guideline.[10] Using this guideline, the following phases are characterized as follows.

Late reproductive phase:[3]
- Changes in menstrual cycle flow/length
- FSH, E2 variable
- AMH and inhibin B will be low
- Some women develop intermittent symptoms.

Menopause transition (perimenopause):
- Increased cycle variability
- FSH increased
- E2 variable
- AMH, inhibin B (low)
  Symptoms of estrogen deficiency, likely.

Postmenopause:
- Cessation of menstruation
- FSH elevated [18,19]
- E2, AMH, inhibin B low, progesterone continually low
  Symptoms of estrogen are much more likely.

Androgens and the Menopause

Androgens are produced by the adrenal cortex and the ovaries. Circulating blood levels of total and free testosterone, dehydroepiandrosterone (DHEA), DHEA sulphate and androstenedione decline with age, this decline commences in the late reproductive years **(Table 2)**. There is no acute change in androgens across the natural menopause.

Surgical menopause is associated with a significant reduction in testosterone and lower androgens have been reported in women with POI.

Though menopause and its effects are actually physiological events in a woman's life, the undesirable effects, which may reach pathological proportions could be mitigated and managed by appropriate preventive measures, early detection, and proper treatment.

TABLE 2: Endocrine changes after menopause.

Increase in	Decrease in
• FSH	• Estrogen (mainly estradiol)
• LH	• Inhibin A
• Estrone:Estradiol	• Inhibin B
• Androgen:Estrogen	• AMH
• Activin	• SHBG
• Cortisol	• Testosterone
	• Androstenedione
	• DHEA

(AMH: anti-Müllerian hormone; DHEA: dehydroepiandrosterone; FSH: follicle-stimulating hormone; LH: luteinizing hormone; SHBG: sex hormone-binding globulin)

■ KEY MESSAGES

- Menopause is a normal physiologic event, defined as the FMP (final menstruation period) and reflecting loss of ovarian follicular function.
- Spontaneous or natural menopause is recognized retrospectively after 12 months of amenorrhea. It occurs at an average age of 51 years, but the age of natural menopause can vary widely.
- Induced menopause refers to the cessation of menstruation that occurs after either bilateral oophorectomy or iatrogenic ablation of ovarian function (e.g., by chemotherapy or pelvic radiation).
- Reproductive aging is associated with marked changes in endocrine functions, mainly in gonadotropins and ovarian hormones.
- Early decrease in inhibin B and AMH heralds reducing ovarian reserve which is followed by high FSH and LH and varying estrogen concentration resulting in irregular menstrual cycles and menopausal symptoms during menopausal transition.
- Adrenal changes concurrent with the menopause transition include elevations in serum cortisol and transient elevations in dehydroepiandrosterone sulfate, androstenediol, and other adrenal androgens.
- Understanding sex steroid receptor function, facilitates development of pharmacologic agents that selectively manipulate these receptors and affect a diverse array of clinical outcomes.
- Menopause due to estrogen deficiency may produce symptoms such as vasomotor symptoms, menstrual irregularities, musculoskeletal disorder, osteoporosis, genitourinary syndrome, and psychosocial and cognitive disorder.
- Primary ovarian insufficiency (POI) describes a transient or permanent loss of ovarian function leading to amenorrhea in women aged younger than 40 years. This condition affects approximately 1% of women. Early menopause describes menopause occurring in women

aged 40–45 years and is experienced by approximately 5% of women. Premature menopause can be used to refer to definitive cases of menopause before the age of 40 years, such as with the surgical removal of both ovaries.
- By the year 2030, the number of postmenopausal women is expected to rise more than 1,200 billion worldwide.
- Healthy aging is about creating the environments and opportunities that enable women to be and do what they value throughout their lives. Taking a few precautions and preventive measures all of us can experience healthy aging.
- Therefore healthcare providers must have wide knowledge regarding the overview of menopause and they must acquire enough updated information to provide optimum treatment to improve the quality-of-life and help in healthy aging of menopause women.

■ REFERENCES

1. Taffe JR, Dennerstein L. Menstrual patterns leading to the final menstrual period. Menopause. 2002;9(1):32-40.
2. Miro F, Parker SW, Aspinall LJ, Coley J, Perry PW, Ellis JE, et al. Origins and consequences of the elongation of the human menstrual cycle during the menopausal transition: the FREEDOM Study. J Clin Endocrinol Metab. 2004;89:4910-5.
3. Harlow SD, Gass M, Hall JE, Lobo R, Maki P, Rebar RW, et al. Executive summary of the Stages of Reproductive Aging Workshop + 10: addressing the unfinished agenda of staging reproductive aging. J Clin Endocrinol Metab. 2012;97:1159-68.
4. Freeman EW, Sammel MD, Gracia CR, Kapoor S, Lin H, Liu L, et al. Follicular phase hormone levels and menstrual bleeding status in the approach to menopause. Fertil Steril. 2005;83:383-5.
5. Burger HG, Hale GE, Dennerstein L, Robertson DM. Cycle and hormone changes during perimenopause: the key role of ovarian function. Menopause. 2008;15:603-12.
6. Burger HG. Unpredictable endocrinology of the menopause transition: clinical, diagnostic and management implications. Menopause Int. 2011;17:153-4.
7. Bromberger JT, Schott LL, Kravitz HM, Sowers M, Avis NE, Gold EB, et al. Longitudinal change in reproductive hormones and depressive symptoms across the menopausal transition: results from the Study of Women's Health Across the Nation (SWAN). Arch Gen Psychiatry. 2010;67:598-607.
8. McKinlay SM, Brambilla DJ, Posner JG. The normal menopause transition. Maturitas. 1992;14(2):103-15.
9. Gold EB, Colvin A, Avis N, Bromberger J, Greendale GA, Powell L, et al. Longitudinal analysis of the association between vasomotor symptoms and race/ethnicity across the menopausal transition: study of women's health across the nation. Am J Public Health. 2006;96:1226-35.
10. Woods NF, Mitchell ES. Symptoms during the perimenopause: prevalence, severity, trajectory, and significance in women's lives. Am J Med. 2005;118(Suppl 12B):14-24.
11. Dennerstein L, Dudley EC, Hopper JL, Guthrie JR, Burger HG. A prospective population-based study of menopausal symptoms. Obstet Gynecol. 2000;96(3):351-8.

12. Soules MR, Sherman S, Parrott E, Rebar R, Santoro N, Utian W, et al. Executive summary: Stages of Reproductive Aging Workshop (STRAW). Fertil Steril. 2001;76:874-8.
13. Kronenberg F. Hot flashes: epidemiology and physiology. Ann N Y Acad Sci. 1990; 592:52-86.
14. Freedman RR, Roehrs TA. Sleep disturbance in menopause. Menopause. 2007; 14(5):826-9.
15. Sarrel PM. Ovarian hormones and vaginal blood flow: using laser Doppler velocimetry to measure effects in a clinical trial of post-menopausal women. Int J Impot Res. 1998;10(Suppl 2):S91-3.
16. Woodard GA, Brooks MM, Barinas-Mitchell E, Mackey RH, Matthews KA, Sutton-Tyrrell K. Lipids, menopause, and early atherosclerosis in Study of Women's Health Across the Nation Heart women. Menopause. 2011;18:376-84.
17. Dugan SA, Powell LH, Kravitz HM, Everson Rose SA, Karavolos K, Luborsky J. Musculoskeletal pain and menopausal status. Clin J Pain. 2006;22(31):325-31.
18. van Disseldorp J, Faddy MJ, Themmen AP, de Jong FH, Peeters PH, van der Schouw YT, et al. Relationship of serum antimüllerian hormone concentration to age at menopause. J Clin Endocrinol Metab. 2008;93(6):2129-34.
19. Hall JE. Neuroendocrine physiology of the early and late menopause. Endocrinol Metab Clin North Am. 2004;33(4):637-59.

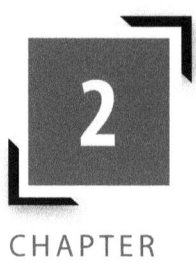

CHAPTER 2

How to Diagnose Menopause?

■ INTRODUCTION

The menopausal transition, or perimenopause, begins on average 4 years before the final menstrual period (FMP) and includes a number of physiologic changes that may affect a woman's quality-of-life. It is characterized by irregular menstrual cycles and marked hormonal fluctuations, often accompanied by hot flushes, sleep disturbances, mood symptoms, and vaginal dryness.[1-6]

The diagnosis of menopause is mostly straightforward if a woman is over the age of 45 years and reports cessation of menstruation for over 12 months, with or without symptoms. The menopause is a clinical diagnosis. The exact age of menopause varies from country-to-country and depends upon environmental and genetic factors. The diagnosis is based on symptoms alone in women without a uterus. If a woman has had a hysterectomy and has classic menopausal symptoms, treatment can be instituted without a firm diagnosis, as menstrual bleeding is not an issue if estrogen is to be prescribed.

Challenging situations, in terms of diagnosis, include women who have had an endometrial ablation, have a progestin-releasing intrauterine device (IUD), are using systemic hormonal contraception (estrogen plus progestin oral, transdermal, or women using implanted/depot progestin). Women have symptoms of menopause but age less than 40 years old, need special attention. This condition is known as premature ovarian insufficiency (POI).

For women under age 40 years: Women in this age group with a change in intermenstrual interval and menopausal symptoms should not be diagnosed with either the menopausal transition or menopause. They have primary ovarian insufficiency (premature ovarian failure). The biology and natural history are of these women are different from natural menopause women. Their etiology and pathogenesis are different and need intensive investigations.

■ EVALUATION

The evaluation for women of all ages should start with an assessment of the woman's menstrual cycle history (ideally with a menstrual calendar) and a detailed history of any menopausal symptoms (hot flushes, sleep disturbances, depression, and vaginal dryness). All women particularly with the symptoms of vaginal dryness, dyspareunia, or sexual dysfunction

should have a pelvic examination to evaluate for vaginal atrophy or for other causes. In general, the symptoms could be:
- Irregular periods, absent periods, heavy bleeding (during perimenopause)
- Hot flushes, night sweats leading to poor sleep
- Tiredness, mood changes/low mood/anxiety/irritability
- Poor self-esteem, poor body image
- Vaginal dryness, decreased sex drive
- Repeated urinary tract infections (UTIs)
- Changes in skin and hair
- Joint pains
- Bloating.

Longer-term problems such as osteoporosis and increase in cardiovascular disease (CVD) appear late. Many symptoms occur before the final cessation of menstruation, i.e., during perimenopause period.

■ PERIMENOPAUSAL SYMPTOMS

Because hormone levels fluctuate during the perimenopausal years, women might present with symptoms of relative estrogen excess, estrogen deficiency or both. Typical estrogen excess symptoms include breast tenderness, menorrhagia, migraine, nausea, shorter cycle length and a shorter follicular phase.[7]

■ THE SYMPTOMS OF THE MENOPAUSE

There is substantial variability between women in the symptoms that occur due to the hormonal changes at menopause. The symptoms listed here are primarily due to systemic estrogen deficiency and most of these are alleviated by estrogen therapy. Common symptoms are:
- *Vasomotor symptoms (VMS)*:
  - Hot flushes
  - Night sweats.
- *Psychological*:
  - Depressive symptoms
  - Anxiety/irritability
  - Sleep disturbance
  - Overall diminished well-being
  - Lessened memory
  - Lessened concentration.
- *General physical*:
  - Sleep disturbance
  - Fatigue
  - Headaches
  - Muscle/joint pains
  - Crawling sensations on skin (formication).

TABLE 1: Menopausal symptoms categorized by guideline NICE, 2016.

Category	Symptoms
Vasomotor	Hot flushes, sweats
Musculoskeletal	Joint and muscle pain
Mood	Low mood
Urogenital	Vaginal dryness
Sexual	Low sexual desire

- *Urogenital and sexual*:
  - Vaginal itching, burning
  - Dryness and dyspareunia
  - Urinary frequency, urgency.

NICE Guidelines, 2016 (Menopausal Symptoms)

The menopausal symptoms according to the National Institute for Health and Care Excellence guidelines, 2016 are given in **Table 1**.

Many women may develop evidences of following health changes:
- *Metabolic*:
  - Central abdominal fat deposition (even in slim women)
  - Insulin resistance and increased risk of type 2 diabetes.
- *Cardiovascular*:
  - Impaired endothelial function (impaired vascular integrity)
  - Increased cholesterol (total cholesterol and low density lipoprotein cholesterol).
- *Skeletal*:
  - Accelerated bone loss
  - Increased fracture risk.
- *Neurological*: Persistent controversy as to whether the fall in estrogen at menopause and decline in androgens with age adversely affect cognitive performance.
- *Urogenital*: Atrophic vulvovaginitis.

Therefore a detailed history taking, physical examination, and vaginal examination need to be performed.

■ MEASUREMENT OF HORMONES: WHEN AND WHY?

Hormonal tests should not routinely be used for diagnosis of the menopause. In particular, the follicle-stimulating hormone (FSH) test is not inappropriate for women taking combined hormonal contraception or a high-dose progestogen, nor should it be used for women aged over 45 years. Blood levels of FSH fluctuate markedly during the years leading up to menopause and they therefore do not help when forming what is actually a clinical diagnosis. The NICE "do not do" list also includes measuring anti-Müllerian hormone (an indicator of ovarian reserve), inhibin A or B (which inhibits FSH production), estradiol, antral follicle count and ovarian volume. However, an FSH test should be considered for women aged 40-45 years with menopausal symptoms, including a change in their menstrual cycle, and in women under the age of 40 years when the menopause is suspected, in whom premature ovarian insufficiency is a possibility.

Hormone measurements are required: To diagnose POI—diagnosis requires FSH to be elevated on at least two occasions and it should be at least 4-6 weeks apart. Where the level should be >25 IU/L and the estradiol level will be low. More investigations are usually indicated once POI is diagnosed.

Other Biochemical Investigations Based on Clinical Assessment

We need to exclude other causes of amenorrhea in younger women such as:
- Pregnancy
- Hyperprolactinemia
- Thyroid disease
- Hypothalamic amenorrhea (anorexia nervosa, etc.).

Also need to exclude other common causes of fatigue, mood change, and hotness:
- *Thyroid disease*: Thyroid stimulating hormone (TSH)
- *Iron deficiency*: Hemoglobin/iron stores
- *Type 2 diabetes*: Fasting blood glucose.

We also need to consider whether fasting lipids, vitamin D measurement required.

■ SYMPTOM PREVALENCE

It is well-established that menopausal symptoms may range from none at all through to debilitating.

VMS are most commonly reported in the late menopause transition and after menopause. VMS are more common in obese women.

Within the US population, symptoms are more common in African-American women than Caucasian women, and less common in Chinese and Japanese women.[8]

High rates of sleeping difficulty, VMS, joint and muscular discomfort and of vaginal dryness have been reported for women living in urban and remote regions across the globe, dispelling the myth that menopausal symptoms are phenomena of the developed world.[9-12]

■ SYMPTOM DURATION

There is no age limit at which menopausal symptoms cease. Women who experience severe symptoms, either from early in the menopause transition or from their final menstrual period, continue to experience severe symptoms for several years.[13]

At least 10% of women have bothersome VMS 10 years after their menopause has occurred, with as many as 16% of 85-year-old continuing to experience VMS.[14] Urogenital atrophy due to estrogen deficiency persists unless treated, so effectively all untreated postmenopausal women are affected.

Women may present with symptoms of metabolic syndrome. The fall in E2 at menopause has a number of adverse metabolic effects and health effects.

After diagnosis of menopause women should know all information and advice about how the menopause progresses, its common symptoms and the long-term health implications. They should be informed about lifestyle changes, diet, exercise, and interventions that could improve their general health and well-being, and the benefits and risks of treatment. The treatments of main interest are menopause hormone therapy. Women in the perimenopausal and 1 year of postmenopausal stages should be offered information about contraception in line with advice for the over 40s from the Faculty of Sexual and Reproductive Healthcare (FSRH).[7] Women who are likely to experience a surgical or medical menopause, e.g., due to cancer therapy, should receive support and information beforehand and be offered referral to a healthcare professional with expertise in the menopause.

■ KEY MESSAGES

- Most women do not need to have any hormonal tests done to diagnose menopause. History of 12 months amenorrhea in a woman after the age of 45 years mostly indicates natural menopause.
- For women using systemic hormonal contraception, hormonal tests are completely uninformative as ovarian function is suppressed. The only way to ascertain a woman's menopausal status while using systemic hormonal contraception is to cease usage.
- The menopausal transition, or perimenopause, begins on average 4 years before the FMP and is marked by irregular menstrual cycles, intense hormonal fluctuations, often accompanied by vasomotor complaints, sleep disturbances, and changes in sexual function.
- The early menopausal transition is characterized by a change in intermenstrual interval, an increase in serum FSH, and normal or high estradiol. The late transition is characterized by more dramatic menstrual cycle changes and greater FSH and estradiol variability.
- Amenorrhoeic women with progestogen IUD in situ—it can usually be treated with estrogen if symptomatic without any diagnostic blood tests needed.
- Endometrial ablation—still need to prescribe progestogen protection for the endometrium. It is appropriate to institute treatment if the woman is symptomatic without any hormonal tests.

- Hot flushes are the most common symptom in perimenopausal women. They are most common in the late menopausal transition and early postmenopausal stage. Hot flushes are often associated with sleep disturbances.
- Genitourinary atrophy symptoms, including vaginal dryness, dyspareunia, and sometimes sexual dysfunction, are most prevalent during the late menopausal transition and postmenopausal years.
- It is considered the gold standard for characterizing reproductive aging from the reproductive years through menopause and includes criteria for the reproductive years, the menopausal transition, perimenopause, FMP, and postmenopause with its symptoms.
- Women between the ages of 40 and 45 years who present with irregular menstrual cycles and menopausal symptoms may be in the menopausal transition. However, for women in this age group, with or without menopausal symptoms, we recommend the same endocrine evaluation as for any woman with oligo-amenorrhea—serum human chorionic gonadotropin (hCG), prolactin, TSH, and FSH.
- For women under age 40 years with irregular menses and menopausal symptoms, women need a complete evaluation for premature ovarian failure.

REFERENCES

1. Taffe JR, Dennerstein L. Menstrual patterns leading to the final menstrual period. Menopause. 2002;9:32-40.
2. Miro F, Parker SW, Aspinall LJ, Coley J, Perry PW, Ellis JE, et al. Origins and consequences of the elongation of the human menstrual cycle during the menopausal transition: the FREEDOM Study. J Clin Endocrinol Metab. 2004;89:4910-5.
3. Harlow SD, Gass M, Hall JE, Lobo R, Maki P, Rebar RW, et al. Executive summary of the Stages of Reproductive Aging Workshop + 10: addressing the unfinished agenda of staging reproductive aging. J Clin Endocrinol Metab. 2012;97:1159-68.
4. Freeman EW, Sammel MD, Gracia CR, Kapoor S, Lin H, Liu L, et al. Follicular phase hormone levels and menstrual bleeding status in the approach to menopause. Fertil Steril. 2005;83:383-92.
5. Burger HG, Hale GE, Dennerstein L, Robertson DM. Cycle and hormone changes during perimenopause: the key role of ovarian function. Menopause. 2008;15: 603-12.
6. Burger HG. Unpredictable endocrinology of the menopause transition: clinical, diagnostic and management implications. Menopause Int. 2011;17:153-4.
7. Randolph JF Jr, Sowers M, Gold EB, Mohr BA, Luborsky J, Santoro N, et al. Reproductive hormones in the early menopausal transition: relationship to ethnicity, body size, and menopausal status. J Clin Endocrinol Metab. 2003;88:1516-22.
8. Manson JM, Sammel MD, Freeman EW, Grisso JA. Racial differences in sex hormone levels in women approaching the transition to menopause. Fertil Steril. 2001; 75:297-304.
9. Gold EB, Colvin A, Avis N, Bromberger J, Greendale GA, Powell L, et al. Longitudinal analysis of the association between vasomotor symptoms and race/ethnicity across the menopausal transition: Study of Women's Health Across the Nation. Am J Public Health. 2006;96:1226-35.

10. Randolph JF Jr, Sowers M, Bondarenko I, Gold EB, Greendale GA, Bromberger JT, et al. The relationship of longitudinal change in reproductive hormones and vasomotor symptoms during the menopausal transition. J Clin Endocrinol Metab. 2005;90:6106-12.
11. Thurston RC, Joffe H. Vasomotor symptoms and menopause: findings from the Study of Women's Health across the Nation. Obstet Gynecol Clin North Am. 2011;38:489-501.
12. Bromberger JT, Assmann SF, Avis NE, Schocken M, Kravitz HM, Cordal A, et al. Persistent mood symptoms in a multiethnic community cohort of pre- and perimenopausal women. Am J Epidemiol. 2003;158:347-56.
13. Su HI, Sammel MD, Freeman EW, Lin H, DeBlasis T, Gracia CR. Body size affects measures of ovarian reserve in late reproductive age women. Menopause. 2008;15:857-61.
14. Greendale GA, Derby CA, Maki PM. Perimenopause and cognition. Obstet Gynecol Clin North Am. 2011;38:519-35.

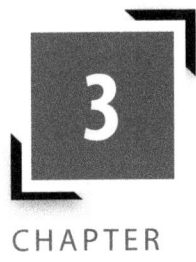

Nutrition, Exercise and Lifestyle for Menopause Women

CHAPTER 3

■ NUTRITION

Optimum nutrition is important determinant of healthy aging. Menopause can occur naturally as part of the normal aging process or abruptly after the surgical removal of the uterus and/or ovaries.[1]

Both obesity and under nutrition in menopause women are significant medical problems. Healthy aging needs optimum nutrition. Every woman has to face this "change of life" at the time of her last period. On an average, women reach menopause at age 51, but it can happen earlier or later. Menopausal women may suffer from symptoms include—hot flushes, night sweats, mood changes, vulvovaginal atrophy, bodyache, and so on. However, some women go through menopause with no real symptoms. Main concerns of menopause are the late consequence, such as osteoporosis, cardiovascular diseases, forgetfulness, metabolic syndrome, and other chronic diseases. But ideal nutrition, exercise, modification of lifestyle may prevent or delay the emergence of these complications.

Longevity of women life is increased (women 73.3 years in Bangladesh) though age of menopause is not changed. By 2030, the World Health Organization (WHO) estimates that the number of menopause women will rise to 1.2 billion women.[1] So, this huge population should lead healthy life, otherwise this will be the burden to the family, nation and that for the society. But for which they need to be fit beyond menopause and so they must adopt preventive strategies to maintain health since their midlife. During midlife, metabolic and hormonal changes occur that impact health and quality-of-life for women. These changes help explain the increased prevalence of chronic diseases observed in postmenopausal women, such as obesity, cardiovascular disease, type 2 diabetes, breast cancer and other reproductive cancers, osteoporosis, osteoarthritis, and autoimmune disorders.[2] As midlife takes women toward menopause, lifestyle behaviors, such as nutrition and physical activity during this phase, may help to prevent the upcoming health challenges.[3,4]

During menopause low calorie requirement, less physical activity, more sedentary habits negatively impact body metabolism, potentially leading to *weight gain*. Estrogen deficiency related to abdominal adiposity. These changes may also affect cholesterol levels and affect the digestion of carbohydrate. Compared with younger women, midlife women have a lower total daily energy (calorie) requirement.[5] This reduction may be associated with a decrease in leisure time physical activity, a gradual loss of lean body mass, and the absence of the increased energy expenditure previously occurring during the luteal phase or second half of the menstrual cycle (i.e., from ovulation to the beginning of the next menstrual period).

Energy intake should be balanced with physical activity to manage body weight. Because requirements for several nutrients, such as calcium, magnesium, vitamin D, and vitamin B6 increase with aging[6-8] this situation results in the challenge of reducing energy (calorie) intake but requiring more nutrients. Thus, menopause women should focus on *nutrient-dense food that is lower in energy (calories)*. To avoid weight gain during the menopause transition, the North American Menopause Society (NAMS) recommends that midlife women should incorporate a daily calorie deficit diet, physical activity and embrace a low-fat diet, and consume more fruits and vegetables.[9]

Many women experience symptoms such as hot flushes, difficulty in sleeping, irritability, forgetfulness, bones pain, genitourinary symptoms, and cardiovascular diseases during this transition period. Additionally, hormone changes lead to declined bone density, which can increase the risk of fractures. Fortunately, making changes in diet may help to relieve menopause symptom and prevent adverse consequences of menopause.

■ NUTRITIONAL NEEDS

Nutritional requirements change with age. After the menopause, overall management should incorporate nutritional recommendations to promote optimal health and well-being. The Dietary Guidelines for Americans 2010 provide guidance to achieve and maintain a healthy body weight, promote health, and prevent chronic diseases.[10] The guidelines emphasize three main points:

1. Balancing energy intake with physical activity to maintain body weight.
2. Consuming more fruits, vegetables, whole grains, fat-free and low-fat dairy products, and sea food.
3. Consuming less food with sodium and saturated fats.

Similar to the DGAC 2010, the American Heart Association (AHA) recommends that women should consume a diet rich in fruits and vegetables; choose whole-grain high-fiber food; consume oily fish at least twice a week; limit intake of saturated fat, cholesterol, alcohol, sodium, and sugar and avoid transfatty acids.

Recommendations for macronutrient distribution of the diet are the same for all healthy women.[5] Midlife and menopause women should be encouraged to substitute saturated and trans-fatty acids with monounsaturated and omega-3 fatty acids. Because the strongest dietary determinants of *elevated LDL cholesterol* concentrations are dietary *saturated fat* and *trans fat*, intakes should be less than 7% and 1% of total energy, respectively.

TABLE 1: Energy requirement of moderately active women.

Age (year)	Women (kcal)
40–44	2,090
50–59	1,980
60–69	1,760

Protein-derived energy should come from fish, poultry, legumes, and low-fat dairy products (good sources of calcium and vitamin D). Fish, especially oily fish, should be included in the diet to get sources of omega-3 fatty acids and reduce the risk of heart disease. Added sugars and refined grains should be limited because they may increase triglyceride concentrations, decrease high-density lipoprotein cholesterol amount.

Nutrition refers to the balance of nutrients taken into the body versus the body's requirement.

■ NUTRITIONAL RECOMMENDATIONS

Good nutrition is important for maintaining or improving overall health as well as reducing the risks of cardiovascular disease and osteoporosis. Nutritional requirements vary from person to person. However, general guidelines suggest that menopause women should strive to consume between 1.5 and 2 cups of fruit each day, between 2 and 2.5 cups of vegetables, and 3 cups of low-fat milk products. They should eat approximately 5-6 oz of grains each day (with a minimum of 3 oz coming from whole grains), and between 5 and 5.5 oz of meat/beans. Plant oils like extra-virgin olive oil, avocados, seeds, and nuts, are also an essential part of a healthy diet and have been found to help prevent diseases.[11] Women should limit the intake of high calorie or sugary drinks as well as alcoholic drinks. They should be consumed in moderation, or not at all. It is recommended that women limit alcohol intake to a maximum of one drink per day (i.e., 12 fl. oz beer, 5 fl. oz wine, or 1.5 fl. oz 80-proof distilled spirits).[12] Good thing is that, Bangladeshi women have fewer tendencies to drink alcohol.

To give advice for nutrition, actually we need to formulate the total requirement of calorie for the particular woman. The US National Academy of Sciences recommends the daily intake, which is given in **Table 1**.

Our women are shorter and having lower body mass index (BMI) than those American women so we may reduce the overall calorie intake in our perspective. So we need to follow:
- Estimating energy/calorie requirement of the particular woman
- Estimating protein requirement [0.8–1 g/kg of adjusted ideal body weight (AIBW) or 20–25% of daily energy requirement]
- Estimating fat requirement (20–25% of daily energy requirement)
- Estimating carbohydrates requirement (supplementation of energy requirement about 45–50% of daily energy requirement)

- Determining food rations
- Dividing daily rations into meals
- Planning a menu (4–5 meals daily).

The followed low energy diet should also be a high fiber diet and eliminate high glycemic index (GI < 75) foods. An optimal number of meals are 4–5 meals a day every 3 hours.[13]

Daily protein intake should not be lower than 0.8 g/kg of adjusted ideal body weight. It should be noted that saturated fats ought to provide less than 7% of energy, polyunsaturated fats of n-6 linoleic acid almost 8% of energy, and of omega n-3 about 2% of energy. The remaining amount of consumed fat should include monounsaturated fats (n-9). Carbohydrates supplement the diet, yet their amount should not be less than 130 g/day.[14] Fiber supply should be within 20–30 g daily, and soluble fiber should constitute 25% of it. During the diet, it is recommended to drink 2 L of still water. In addition, table salt intake should be limited to 5 g/day.[15,16] Supply of vitamins and minerals should be adequate.

At a glance dietary recommendation of women after menopause is following (Consensus Conference convened by the US National Institutes of Health of 1994):

- Total fat intake <30% of daily calories
- Daily fiber intake of 20–30 mg
- Diet should contain variety of fruits, vegetables and whole-grain cereals
- Daily calcium intake of 1,200 mg without at least half of it should come from dietary source
- Daily vitamin D intake should contain 800 IU/day.

Although saturated fats are to be avoided, omega-3 fatty acids are recommended because they have been linked to improve cardiac function and diabetes prevention. Monounsaturated fats are approved.

ESSENTIAL NUTRIENTS

Women going through the menopause should increase their intake of food sources of calcium, magnesium and vitamins D and K to maintain the integrity of the skeleton. In addition, high amounts of phosphorous, found in red meat, processed foods and fizzy drinks, should also be avoided. Too much phosphorous in the diet accelerates the loss of minerals such as calcium and magnesium from the bone. Reducing sodium, caffeine and protein from animal products can also help the body to maintain calcium stores.

Women need to eat foods high in magnesium and boron. These are minerals, which are important for the replacement of bone and thus help to reduce the risk of osteoporosis. Apples, pears, grapes, dates, raisins, legumes and nuts are good sources of boron. Other vitamins and minerals that are vital for bone health are magnesium, vitamin E, vitamin D, and zinc.

Numerous studies have attested to the value of folic acid, vitamin C, vitamin E, calcium, and vitamin D for general health as well as prevention of some specific disease processes, such as colorectal cancer, cardiovascular disease, and osteoporosis. Dietary supplements can be appropriately incorporated into the overall nutrition plan to ensure that women receive sufficient amounts of these nutrients. Specific minimal daily requirements vary depending on the country or organization issuing.

Folic acid has been linked to primary prevention of coronary heart disease (CHD) and colorectal cancer.

Vitamin C is an antioxidant that has been associated with a reduced prevalence of CHD and stroke, as well as cancer in some studies. Vitamin E is also an antioxidant that has been associated with a reduced risk of nonfatal myocardial infarction, but not cardiovascular or total mortality. Vitamin E may also relieve hot flushes. However, it can increase bleeding disorders if combined with anticoagulants (associated with mega doses of vitamin E > 800 IU/day). Vitamin A is required for healthy skin and mucous membranes, but there has been no consensus about its possible role in preventing cancer. Furthermore, high levels of intake were associated with low bone density and increased risk of hip fractures in one study. Vitamin D has antiproliferative effects, and intake of this nutrient shows an inverse relationship with the risk of colorectal cancer. Vitamin D also stimulates the absorption of calcium. Calcium delays the rate of bone loss. Calcium also lowers the risk of colon cancer and hypertension. Average daily requirement (US National Academy of Sciences) is as follows:

- Folic acid—400 ng
- Vitamin C—60 µg
- Vitamin E—30 IU
- Calcium—1,500 mg
- Fiber—20-30 g.

Dietary fiber has been associated with a reduced risk of CHD and related mortality, but has no protective effect against colorectal cancer or adenoma. Omega-3 fatty acids have the potential benefits of lowering triglyceride levels, preventing cardiac arrhythmias, preventing thrombogenesis, and improving arterial compliance.

■ EXERCISE

Physical exercise provides potential health and fitness benefits for women of all ages, especially for midlife women and beyond.[17,18] After the cessation of menses, exercise can confer many of the benefits. Aerobic exercise improves carbohydrate metabolism, improves the lipid profile, reduces blood pressure, and may reduce the rate of bone loss.

Soon after menopause women start loosing bone mass. Therefore, it is very important to adopt the strategies to prevent further bone loss. Weight-bearing exercises maintain or increase bone density while increasing flexibility, endurance and strength. Sedentary lifestyle increases the risk of breast cancer and increases bone loss. Exercise improves the bone remodeling and reduces bone resorption.

More active women tend to be leaner than inactive peers, physical activity may slow the rate of change in weight across time and with menopause, and physical activity may protect against the development of obesity.[19]

For the prevention of cardiovascular disease, midlife women should be encouraged to accumulate at least 150 min/week of moderate exercise, 75 min/week of vigorous exercise, or an equivalent combination of both.[20] Activity can be performed throughout the day in episodes of at least 10 minutes. Increasing to 300 min/week of moderate-intensity aerobic activity, 150 minutes of vigorous intensity, or a combination of both, can provide additional cardiovascular benefits. A physical activity program should be individualized and also include resistance training or muscle-strengthening exercise, this exercise should include each major muscle group 2 to 3 days/week.[21]

Osteoporosis is a major risk of fracture so the NAMS also recommends that women should be encouraged to engage in regular physical activity, avoid smoking, and limit alcohol intake.[9] Thus, a healthy lifestyle should be followed by menopause women to prevent adverse effects on bone health. The ACSM Position Stand "Physical Activity and Bone Health" points out two strategies to make the skeleton more resistant to fracture: (1) to maximize the gain in bone mineral density in the first three decades of life and (2) to minimize the decline in bone mineral density after age of 40 years.[22] Weight-bearing and strength training exercises are recommended as strategies for bone development and maintenance.[23] Weight-bearing activities can be as simple as brisk walking (although jogging or running provides impact-loading benefits to the skeleton); resistance training can be accomplished using machines, resistance bands, free weights, or barbells. Physical activity (including balance, leg strength, flexibility and/or endurance training) also is valuable in fracture prevention by reducing the incidence of falls.[22] Exercise improves quality-of-life in addition to the previously documented benefits of exercise and physical activity; both cross-sectional research and interventional research demonstrate positive changes in quality-of-life for physically active midlife and menopause women.[24,25] Physical activity is also associated with higher levels of well-being, positive mood, and vigor and lower depression, anxiety, and perceived stress in mid-life women.[19,24] Given the many areas of potential positive impact, health and fitness professionals should encourage women to exercise regularly throughout their life-spans. Physical activity in the form of a complete balanced exercise program

(including cardiorespiratory, resistance, flexibility, and neuromotor training) is the key for health promotion and disease prevention:
- *Weight control*:
  - If BMI is 20-23 kg/m^2, and waist circumference <80 cm woman is perfect. She just needs to maintain her optimum weight.
  - If overweight, the aim is to achieve a weight reduction of at least 5-10% of weight in 6-12 months.
  - Physical exercise and dietary modification may help to achieve desired weight.
- *Psychosocial approaches*: Regular mental stimulation, continuing employment, engaging in social activity help to develop a positive self-image.
- *Education*: Education on menopause, its implications and symptoms, gynecological and medical problems that increase in the postmenopausal period, sexual health, coping with psychological dilemma, screening of discuses malignancy an healthy lifestyle practices.

Health and fitness of menopausal women is most important to help to gain maximum health benefits while reducing the risk of chronic disease. Menopause women should be encouraged to adopt a healthy lifestyle, including regular physical activity and a nutritious diet, while avoiding cigarette smoking and overuse of alcohol. It should be started from midlife or from perimenopuse. Women should focus on getting more nutrients and fewer calories by consuming a diet rich in fruits and vegetables, whole grains, and high-fiber food.

KEY MESSAGES

- Proper nutrition is essential for maintaining overall health and reducing the risk of cardiovascular disease, osteoporosis and other chronic diseases after the cessation of menses.
- Dietary recommendations include restricting fat intake, ensuring adequate fiber intake, and consuming a varied diet including fresh fruits, vegetables, whole grains, and proteins.
- Women should avoid sodium, added sugars, saturated/trans-fats red meat, saturated fat, alcohol, too much salt, and smoking.
- Appropriate amounts of essential nutrients (including vitamins C, D and E, calcium, and folic acid) should be provided through diet and/or supplements.
- Daily requirement of calcium 1,200 mg and vitamin D 800 IU is recommended. Half of calcium must be taken from dietary intake and women should get regular sunlight to prevent vitamin D deficiency.
- In general, it would be wise to eat smaller portion more often through the day so as to keep a steady blood sugar level and to prevent sudden cravings. Also diet should contain all of the macronutrients (lean protein,

healthy fats and complex carbohydrates) in a balanced way. Proper hydration is important too.
- Exercise is the corner stone of healthy lifestyle. Along with diet, healthy lifestyle includes regular physical exercise and mental recreation.
- The exercise prescription should be tailored to the individual, based on assessments of cardiovascular fitness, muscular strength and balance.
- Finally menopause women should keep positive attitude and must adopt healthy approaches to be happy and fit.

REFERENCES

1. World Health Organization. Research on the menopause in the 1990s. Report of a WHO Scientific Group. World Health Organ Tech Rep Ser. 1996;866:1-107.
2. Sowers M, Harlow S, Karvonen C. Menopause: Its Epidemiology. Goldman MB, Troisi R, Rexrode KM (Eds). Salt Lake City: Academic Press; 2013. pp. 57.
3. Lambrinoudaki I, Ceasu I, Depypere H, Erel T, Rees M, Schenck-Gustafsson K, et al. EMAS position statement: diet and health in midlife and beyond. Maturitas. 2013;74(1):99-104.
4. Lange-Collett J. Promoting health among perimenopausal women through diet andexercise. J Am Acad Nurse Pract. 2002;14(4):172.
5. National Research Council. Dietary Reference Intakes for Energy, Carbohydrate, Fiber, Fat, Fatty Acids, Cholesterol, Protein, and Amino Acids (Macronutrients). Washington (DC): The National Academies Press; 2005.
6. Institute of Medicine. Dietary Reference Intakes for Calcium and Vitamin D. Washington (DC): The National Academies Press; 2011.
7. Woolf K, Bushman BA, Gabriel KP, Carter S. Healthy Lifestyles in Menopausal Transition. ACSMce Online. 2015:1-9.
8. Institute of Medicine. Dietary Reference Intakes for Calcium, Phosphorus, Magnesium, Vitamin D, and Fluoride. Washington (DC): The National Academies Press; 1997.
9. Shifren JL, Gass ML. NAMS Recommendations for Clinical Care of Midlife Women Working Group. The North American Menopause Society recommendations for clinical care of midlife women. Menopause. 2014;21(10):1038-62.
10. US Department of Agriculture. US Department of Health and Human Services. Dietary Guidelines for Americans, 2010, 7th edition. Washington (DC): US Government Printing Office; 2010.
11. Dietary Guidelines for Americans 2015–2020, 8th edition (2008 Physical Activity Guidelines). [online] Available from: health.gov/dietaryguidelines/2015/guidelines/ [Last accessed February, 2021].
12. Womenshealth.gov. Women's Health. [online] Available from: www.womenshealth.gov/ [Last accessed February, 2021].
13. Jarosz M. Praktyczny podręcznik dietetyki. Warszawa: Instytut Żywności i Żywienia; 2010.
14. Jarosz M. Normy żywienia dla populacji polskiej—nowelizacja. Warszawa: Instytut Żywności i Żywienia; 2012.
15. Białkowska M. Leczenie dietetyczne–ciągle aktualna metoda terapii otyłości. Postępy Nauk Medycznych. 2013;5:38-43.
16. Ciborowska H, Rudnicka A. Żywienie zdrowego i chorego człowieka. Warszawa: Wydawnictwo Lekarskie PZWL; 2012 (Dietetyka).
17. Khan UI, Wang D, Karvonen-Gutierrez CA, Khalil N, Ylitalo KR, Santoro N. Progression from metabolically benign to at-risk obesity in perimenopausal women: a longitudinal analysis of Study of Women Across the Nation (SWAN). J Clin Endocrinol Metab. 2014;99(7):2516-25.

18. Sternfeld B, Bhat AK, Wang H, Sharp T, Quesenberry CP Jr. Women. Med Sci Sports Exerc. 2005;37(7):1195-202.
19. Sternfeld B, Dugan S. Physical activity and health during the menopausal transition. Obstet Gynecol Clin North Am. 2011;38(3):537-66.
20. Mosca L, Benjamin EJ, Berra K, Bezanson JL, Dolor RJ, Lloyd-Jones DM, et al. Effectiveness-based guidelines for the prevention of cardiovascular disease in women—2011 update: a guideline from the American Heart Association. Circulation. 2011;123(11):1243-62.
21. Garber CE, Blissmer B, Deschenes MR, Franklin BA, Lamonte MJ, Lee IM, et al. American College of Sports Medicine position stand. Quantity and quality of exercise for developing and maintaining cardiorespiratory, musculoskeletal, and neuromotor fitness in apparently healthy adults: guidance for prescribing exercise. Med Sci Sports Exerc. 2011;43(7):1334-59.
22. Kohrt WM, Bloomfield SA, Little KD, Nelson ME, Yingling VR. American College of Sports Medicine. American College of Sports Medicine position stand: physical activity and bone health. Med Sci Sports Exerc. 2004;36(11):1985-96.
23. North American Menopause Society. Management of osteoporosis in postmenopausal women: 2010 position statement of The North American Menopause Society. Menopause. 2010;17(1):25-54.
24. Asbury EA, Chandrruangphen P, Collins P. The importance of continued exercise participation in quality of life and psychological well-being in previously inactive postmenopausal women: a pilot study. Menopause. 2006;13(4):561-7.
25. Mansikkamäki K, Raitanen J, Malila N, Sarkeala T, Männistö S, Fredman J, et al. Physical activity and menopause-related quality of life—a population-based cross-sectional study. Maturitas. 2015;80(1):69-74.

CHAPTER 4

Vasomotor Symptoms and Menopause

■ INTRODUCTION

Menopause is the permanent cessation of menstruation; ovaries stop producing estrogen; and may be associated with a wide range of symptoms. Menopause is a normal biological event that affects all women.

Life expectancy for women is increasing worldwide. Therefore, most women can expect to spend a significant portion of their lives in a postmenopausal state and may suffer from menopausal symptoms due to estrogen deficiency. The most common symptoms are vasomotor symptoms (VMS), which include hot flashes (also referred to as hot flushes) and night sweats. Beside VMS, women may suffer from vaginal dryness, sleep disturbances, and osteoporosis in addition to variety of other physical and psychological symptoms.[1] Hot flashes are one of the most common and distressing symptoms associated with menopause, occurring in >75% of postmenopausal women.[2]

Vasomotor symptoms encompass hot flashes, night sweats, feeling of cold, and palpitation. Again, VMS, or hot flashes and night sweats, are often considered the cardinal symptoms of menopause.

Hot flashes present as transient periods of intense heat in the upper body, arms, head, and face, often followed by flushing of the skin and profuse sweating all over the body. VMS can negatively affect the quality-of-life.[3] The prevalence of VMS is varying by geography, socioeconomic, and cultural context.[4] In the USA, over 60% of women have experienced VMS; the figure exceeds 60% in Europe and 50% in Australia. VMS are reported less frequently by Japanese and Chinese women but more frequently by African American women.[5]

Many to most women describe their symptoms as severe, but only approximately 20–30% of women seek medical attention for the treatment.[6-8] Women find VMS as more bothersome, even after accounting for the higher frequency of their VMS. It produces negative effects on their day-to-day activities and quality-of-life. The relationship between negative affect and VMS is not fully understood and may involve a complex interplay between physiologic and psychological factors. It is well-established that negative affect can influence symptom reporting, with a tendency toward elevated symptom reporting in the context of negative affect.[9]

■ MECHANISM

The exact mechanism explaining the emergence of VMS is a mystery; however, evidence points toward a disturbance of the temperature regulating mechanism in the hypothalamus. The disturbances associated with estrogen deprivation render neurotransmitter within the central nervous system unable to maintain body temperature within the optimal range.[10] The thermoneutral zone is narrowed in women with hot flashes.[11] While premenopausal women initiate mechanisms to dissipate heat when the core body temperature increases by 0.4°C, this happens with much lower increase in temperature in menopausal women.[12]

The feeling of warmth results from inappropriate peripheral vasodilatation with increased digital and cutaneous blood flow. Perspiration results in rapid heat loss and a decrease in core body temperature below normal. Shivering may then occur as a normal mechanism to restore the core temperature to normal.[13] Estrogen (E2) administration restores the "thermoneutral zone" to normal and largely abolishes hot flashes. One hypothesis, now supported by increasing evidence, suggests that KNDy (kisspeptin, neurokinin B, and dynorphin) neurons mediate the luteinizing hormone (LH) and thermoregulatory changes.[14] High level of follicle-stimulating hormone (FSH) and low serum concentration of estrogen, testosterone, and progesterone[6] correlate with VMS. Though The Study of Women's Health Across the Nation (SWAN) fails to show any significant association between VMS and serum concentrations of estrogen, testosterone, dehydroepiandrosterone sulfate (DHEAS), sex-hormone binding globulin (SHBG) or with free testosterone index, most research indicating that E2 administration reduces VMS and widens the thermoneutral zone adds support to this treatment.[15] Recently, concern is raised for heart diseases in women suffering from VMS.

Vasomotor symptoms are shown to be associated with increased risk of cardiovascular disease,[16] and great bone loss.[17]

■ RISK FACTORS FOR VASOMOTOR SYMPTOMS

Obesity: Obese postmenopausal women have higher serum estrone concentrations than lean women due to increased peripheral conversion of androstenedione in adipose tissue[18,19] but paradoxically, these women are more likely to have hot flashes.[20,21] Weight loss may help reduce their hot flashes.[22] High BMI and weight gain have been documented as protective[5] and risk factors.[23] BMI did not associate significantly with psychosocial or sexual symptoms at either stage of menopause.[24]

Anxiety, depression, and perceived stress have been associated with increased VMS likelihood.[25] Negative mood has been associated with VMS.[26] VMS and mood appear to be related in numerous and potentially complex ways. However, interestingly many women with VMS do not experience mood disturbances or depression.

Smoking and[20,21] reduced physical activity have not been related to VMS. Romani et al. reported significantly positive relation between physical activity and moderate or severe hot flashes but no relation between hot flash frequency and physical activity.[27] The effects of exercise on VMS are mixed;[28] however, increased physical activity may improve sleep and general well-being.

Socioeconomic factors: Obtaining less than a high school education and having difficulty paying for basics are associated with a higher frequency of hot flashes.[27] Low socioeconomic status has been consistently associated with VMS[28] dispelling the myth that menopausal symptoms are phenomena of the developed world.

Hormonal concentrations: Annual serum FSH levels, but not other hormones (estradiol, testosterone, DHEAS), when collectively modeled longitudinally, are associated with both the prevalence and frequency of VMS.[1]

Ethnic factors: African American women report more frequent hot flashes than Caucasian women, whereas Japanese and Chinese women report less frequent hot flashes.[5]

Genetic variants: Women who have variations in the gene that codes for tachykinin receptor 3 (*TACR3)* are more likely to experience hot flashes than women without those variations.[29]

The role of climate, environment, temperature, and altitude in the development of VMS has not been sufficiently explored. SWAN data found significant positive association between increasing seasonality and hot flashes.[30] The colligative group for research of the climacteric in Latin America found that women living at higher altitude had lower hot flashes, in contrast to UAE, where no association between season variability and hot flashes was found.

■ DURATION OF SYMPTOMS

It varies from woman to woman. There is no age limit at which menopausal symptoms cease. The best estimate of total VMS duration comes from the SWAN study,[31] which showed that the median total VMS duration was 7.4 years, with symptoms persisting for a median of 4.5 years after the final menstrual period. Women who were premenopausal or early perimenopausal when they first experienced VMS had the longest total duration (>11.8). Interestingly, at least 10% of women have bothersome VMS 10 years after their menopause has occurred, with as many as 16% of the 85 year olds continuing to experience VMS.[23]

■ PRESENTATION

Hot flashes typically begin as the sudden sensation of heat centered on the upper chest and face that rapidly becomes generalized. The sensation of heat often lasts from 2 to 4 minutes, is often associated with profuse perspiration and occasionally palpitations, and is sometimes followed by chills, shivering, and a feeling of anxiety. Hot flashes may range from an average of less than one each day to as many as one per hour during the day and night. Studies showed that hot flashes are associated with adverse health indicators such as increased cardiovascular risk and greater bone loss/increased bone turnover.[32,33] So history of any chest pain or bone pain needs to be evaluated thoroughly.

■ SLEEP DISTURBANCE

The optimum amount for a healthy adult is deemed to be around seven hours. Insufficient sleep has been shown to have later detrimental effects on things like our mental health, heart health, cognitive functions and even risk of osteoporosis. Further, too much sleep (more than 8 hours), can be associated with increased risk of cardiovascular disease though cause and effect are unclear; prolonged sleep may be a marker for underlying disease.

Vasomotor symptoms can disrupt sleep in peri- and postmenopausal women. Although VMS is not the only cause of sleep disturbance, it accounts for 27% of wakefulness during the night, the estimated prevalence of difficulty sleeping by studies was 32-40% in the early menopausal transition, increasing to 38-46% in the late transition.[34,35] There are many other issues that disturb sleep in menopause women including primary sleep disorders, anxiety, and depression.

■ HISTORY

Though symptoms of VMS are straightforward, it must include about the differential diagnosis of carcinoid syndrome, medications, hyperthyroidism, history of any infection, and mental disorder. Though symptoms are mainly hot flushes and night sweating, but we need to perform thorough general examination, breast examination, per abdominal examination, and vaginal examination.

■ INVESTIGATIONS

These are mainly done to exclude other causes of night sweat or hot flashes and eligibility for menopause hormone therapy (MHT) as one of the management options is MHT. Usually, complete blood count, postprandial sugar, thyroid hormone, liver function test, transvaginal sonography, and cervical smear are carried out. *All women* should be reviewed in terms of:
- Cardiovascular disease risk (blood pressure and lipids)
- Diabetes (fasting blood glucose)
- Urogenital health (consider local hormonal/nonhormonal therapy)
- Cancer screening—breast examination, PAP smear, and mammogram (recommended frequency varies between countries).

MANAGEMENT

General Principle

It depends upon symptom severity, coexistent diseases, and personal choice. Lifestyle modification is one of the most important measures to alleviate VMS.

Lifestyle Modification

There are many lifestyle changes that can be implemented and should be encouraged to help women to alleviate the VMS associated with menopause. Many women have identified having triggering factors such as alcohol, spicy foods, and hot foods or drinks; simple avoidance of such substances may help to reduce their occurrence. If the patient is a smoker, smoking cessation should strongly be encouraged; other suggestions include lifestyle changes that will help lower or help prevent an increased core body temperature.

Cooling effects can be obtained by followings behavioral measures—women with mild flashes (hot flashes that do not interfere with usual activities) usually do not need pharmacotherapy. Instead, simple behavioral measures such as lowering room temperature, using fans, dressing in layers of clothing that can be easily shed, and avoiding triggers (such as spicy foods and stressful situations) can help to reduce the number of hot flashes. Women need to wear cotton light clothing, use bed fan, cold pack beneath pillow, and maintain low ambient temperature at home. Other potential options may include weight loss, cognitive behavioral therapy (CBT), vitamin E, and hypnosis.

Pharmacotherapy

Menopause hormone therapy is the choice of drug in most women with moderate to very severe hot flashes and having no contraindications. Most of the studies proved that MHT could improve hot flashes more effectively than any other interventions. Cochrane review of randomized controlled trials concluded that, for the treatment of VMS, MHT is highly efficacious, with reductions in both frequency and severity in the order of 75% (Alaster H Maclennan; Therapy versus Placebo for hot flushes: Cochrane Database Systemic Rev. 2004;(4):CD002978). Several core recommendations from different menopause societies and international menopause society suggest that—"MHT is the most effective treatment for VMS associated with menopause at any age, but *benefits are more likely to outweigh risks* for symptomatic women before the age of 60 years or within 10 years after menopause".

Women having uterus should use combined MHT, i.e., estrogen with progestin, while those who have undergone hysterectomy can receive estrogen only without progesterone. Progestins are used to prevent endometrial hyperplasia and thereby endometrial carcinoma. Women with premature ovarian insufficiency should be treated with MHT at least until the age of natural menopause. Oral estrogen is associated with an increased risk of venous thromboembolism (VTE), although the absolute risk is small for women <60 years old. The risk appears to be lower/not at all with transdermal estrogen. Therefore, transdermal estrogen is preferred for women at increased risk of VTE, i.e., smokers and obese women. The regimen containing estrogen in women having uterus must use progestin to prevent endometrial hyperplasia or endometrial carcinoma. The following types of progestins regimens can be used:

- Oral micronized *progesterone* (200 mg/day for 12 days) reduces the risk of hyperplasia to the same degree as *medroxyprogesterone acetate* (2.5 mg/day continuously or 10 mg/day for 12 days).
- Lower doses of combined estrogen-progestin therapy [conjugated estrogen (0.3 or 0.45 mg/day) with *medroxyprogesterone acetate* (1.5 or 2.5 mg/day)] also appear to be endometrial protective, and so can be used.
- Levonorgestrel-releasing intrauterine systems (LNG-IUS) are contraceptive agents that have been used for endometrial protection by some peri- and postmenopausal women taking estrogen. The strategy is to avoid the potential excess risk of cardiovascular disease and breast cancer associated with systemic therapy.

Most uniform regimen recommended oral or transdermal estrogen in combination with micronized progesterone at 100 mg daily, or sequential use of 200 mg micronized progesterone 14 days a month can also be employed.

Thorough discussion of risks and benefits of MHT is mandatory to empower women to choose the right treatment. However, for women with a history of breast cancer, coronary heart disease (CHD), a previous VTE or stroke, or those at moderate or high risk for these complications, alternatives to hormone therapy should be discussed and suggested.[36]

Bazedoxifene/Conjugated Estrogen

An emerging class of drugs called tissue selective estrogen complexes (TSECs) involves the combination of a selective estrogen receptor modulator (SERM) and an estrogen.[37] Bazedoxifene, a SERM, combined with conjugated estrogens, is available in the United States and the European Union for the treatment of postmenopausal VMS and osteoporosis prevention,[38] but not yet available in Bangladesh. This combination of conjugated estrogen 0.45 mg/bazedoxifene 20 mg in women with moderate-to-severe hot flashes decreases hot flash frequency by approximately 75% (vs. 50% for placebo).[39] This regimen may avoid side effects of progesterone.

Combination of estrogen plus intrauterine levonorgestrel approach has been suggested as a means of giving estrogen without the systemic effects of a progestogen, while preventing uterine stimulation.[40] Also, it is very effective for having abnormal bleeding, and/or who need contraception at perimenopause age.

Side effects: Common side effects of estrogen include breast soreness, which can often be minimized by using lower doses. Some women experience mood symptoms and bloating with progestin therapy. Vaginal bleeding may occur in women who receive cyclic estrogen–progestin regimens and is common in the early months of a continuous estrogen–progestin regimen, but in most cases, it subsides along with the time. If it persists beyond 6 months, primary evaluation should be carried out.

If the evaluation of postmenopausal bleeding reveals benign causes, MHT can be continued. To avoid bleeding or spotting, switching to a continuous regimen of progestin of MHT solve the problem. However, for women who are newly menopausal, breakthrough bleeding can be anticipated. In that case, continuous progesterone is better. Both oral and vaginal continuous administration of micronized progesterone 100 mg capsules is well-tolerated for most of the women.

The most effective pharmacologic alternatives to estrogen include some of the antidepressants in the selective serotonin reuptake inhibitors (SSRI) and selective norepinephrine reuptake inhibitors (SNRI) classes.[41] Their efficacy has been demonstrated in individual placebo-controlled trials.[42] Although no head-to-head trials have been performed, indirect comparisons suggest that venlafaxine, desvenlafaxine, paroxetine, and citalopram have a similar modest benefit for hot flashes. One author of this topic suggests low-dose paroxetine (7.5 mg/day)[43] as the first choice of SSRI/SNRI, since this is the only agent that has received approval by the US Food and Drug Administration (FDA) for the treatment of hot flashes. Paroxetine preparations shown to be modestly effective for hot flashes include paroxetine mesylate (7.5 mg/day) and paroxetine hydrochloride [10 and 20 mg/day, and 12.5 mg and 25 mg/day (controlled release)].[44] Side effects are nausea, change in bowel habits, decreased libido, dry mouth, and weight gain (not common). Concomitant use of tamoxifen should be avoided in women taking paroxetine.

Effectiveness: FDA approved it to treat hot flashes. It tends to be effective in women who are also suffering with insomnia and vasomotor symptoms. Improvement in hot flashes has been shown in well-designed studies. While SSRIs or SNRIs are preferred as first-line therapy for most women, gabapentin may be a better option in some women, for example, women whose hot flashes are primarily at night and who are the breast cancer survivors.

Side effects: Fatigue, dizziness, nausea, disorientation, swelling, and weight gain.

In a trial comparing venlafaxine and gabapentin, hot flash reduction was similar with both drugs, but patients preferred venlafaxine by a 2:1 ratio.[45]

Clonidine, a centrally active alpha-2 adrenergic agonist, was modestly more effective than placebo in a meta-analysis of 10 trials.[46]

Oxybutynin, an oral anticholinergic agent used primarily for overactive bladder, was more effective than placebo for relief of hot flashes in an observational study, a randomized clinical trial, and a preliminary report from a second clinical trial.[47]

The thermoregulatory center in the hypothalamus is innervated by KNDy neurons that are stimulated by neurokinin B (NKB) and inhibited by estrogen. After menopause, estrogen declines and NKB signaling is increased. It has been proposed that this results in unregulated KNDy neuron activation and VMS.[48] Antagonism of NKB signaling at its receptor [neurokinin 3 receptor (NK3R)] has been studied as an alternative to MHT for management of hot flashes, an approach that appears to be promising.

Tibolone

It reduces VMS when compared with placebo, has a beneficial effect on bone mineral density,[49] and may be more effective than estrogen/progestin therapy for treatment of sexual dysfunction in postmenopausal women.

However, tibolone has been associated with an increased risk of stroke and possibly breast cancer, and it is not recommended in routine use for hot flash management. Some women may have vaginal bleeding/endometrial hyperplasia—while vaginal bleeding with tibolone[14] and the rate of unscheduled bleeding is lower than that for MHT. If tibolone is chosen, it should be administered in women who have passed 1 year of menopause.

Breast Cancer Survivors

Women with breast cancer have more problems with hot flashes than other women for a number of reasons. Aromatase inhibitors may also cause hot flashes, but they tend to be less frequent and less severe.[50]

Though there is no evidence for an increased risk of breast cancer recurrence in women taking strong inhibitors of *CYP2D6* (paroxetine) with tamoxifen, most studies suggest other agents such as citalopram or venlafaxine in this setting.

Cognitive Behavioral Therapy

Cognitive behavioral therapy appears to be a modestly effective intervention for menopause-associated insomnia[51] but less so for hot flashes.[52] A major limitation of CBT is the need for frequent in-person visits.

Hypnosis appears to reduce perceived hot flashes in breast cancer survivors and may have additional benefits such as reduced anxiety and depression and improves sleep.

Mind–Body-based Therapies

Small number of studies of mind-body-based therapies (stress management, relaxation, deep breathing techniques, and guided imagery) had mixed results in two meta-analyses.[53]

Mindfulness training: A randomized trial of mindfulness-based stress reduction (MBSR) reported a decrease in menopausal hot flashes. Though mindfulness training was not shown to be very effective in reducing the hot flash intensity scores (based upon frequency and severity) when compared with no treatment.[54]

Black Cohosh

Among the alternative therapies available for management of hot flashes, black cohosh (*Actaea racemosa* or *Cimicifuga racemosa*) is one of the most widely used.[55] Black cohosh is a popular herbal supplement that is widely used for the management of the VMS associated with menopause. A 2012 Cochrane review of 16 controlled trials did not show any significant improvement of hot flashes. Position statement of North American menopause society. failed to demonstrate a clinical benefit associated with the herbal supplement.[52]

Acupuncture

Acupuncture is among the most frequently used complementary therapies for hot flashes; however, results thus far are conflicting.[56] In a systematic review and meta-analysis, acupuncture was less effective than MHT (three trials), no different from sham acupuncture (eight studies), but statistically more effective than no therapy (four trials).[57]

Flaxseed

Flaxseed is very popular for many years, but it has not been shown to be more effective than placebo for hot flashes.[58]

Exercise

An increasing amount of research is being undertaken on the effect of exercise on hot flashes. However, there is currently no evidence from randomized controlled trials that show that exercise is an effective treatment for hot flashes. But MHT is superior to any treatment for hot flashes. Clinical trials, systematic reviews, and a meta-analysis have not found a significant beneficial effect of exercise on hot flashes.[59,60] Hormone therapy was more effective than exercise in one trial.[61]

Evening primrose oil, Dong quai (*Angelica sinensis*) is a Chinese herb, Ginseng (*Panax ginseng*), and Wild Yam (*Dioscorea villosa*) a natural progesterone are being used to treat vasomotor symptoms and hot flashes.

However, a double-blind, placebo-controlled, cross-over study found no significant difference in menopausal symptoms between these treatment and placebo groups. Isoflavones can be found in soybeans, chickpeas, lentils, and other legumes. Lignans can be found in flaxseed, whole grains, and some fruits and vegetables. Although these foods may be healthy, they have not been proven to be effective in alleviating menopausal symptoms.

Yoga

The symptom assessment was made using the Greene Climacteric Scale and it was reported that there was a decrease in VMS in the group involved in the yoga program.[62]

Stellate Ganglion Block

The positive effect of stellate ganglion block on hot flashes was first reported in a case report by Lipov and colleagues. In trial of 40 patients randomized to 3 months of stellate ganglion blocks or pregabalin therapy, both therapies were effective, but the reduction in hot flashes was greater with stellate ganglion blocks.[63] It is not popular and more studies yet to be required to recommend.

■ KEY MESSAGE

- Vasomotor symptoms or "hot flashes" are the most common complaint during the menopausal transition and beyond, occurring in up to 80% of women.
- Frequent VMS can be disabling, affecting a woman's social life, psychological health, sense of well-being, and ability to work. Women with hot flushes are more likely to experience disturbed sleep, depressive symptoms, and significant reductions in quality-of-life as compared to asymptomatic women.
- The most effective therapy for relieving VMS and reducing their impact on quality-of-life is MHT. However, postmenopausal women with mild hot flashes usually do not seek or require pharmacologic intervention. Simple lifestyle changes and behavioral therapy such as keeping the core body temperature cool are often adequate to manage symptoms.
- Menopause hormone therapies, including estrogens and progestogens, are the most well-known effective agents in relieving hot flashes.
- Nonhormonal prescription drugs, including certain antidepressant agents, SNRI, SSRI, gabapentin, and clonidine, may afford some relief from hot flashes. These alternatives can be considered when hormone therapy is contraindicated or not desired.
- A woman should know all the options with the risks and benefits to alleviate her symptoms so that she is able to improve her quality-of-life and prevent the long-term complications.

■ REFERENCES

1. Woods NF, Mitchell ES. Symptoms during the perimenopause: Prevalence, severity, trajectory, and significance in women's lives. Am J Med. 2005;118:14-24.
2. Couzi R, Helzlsouer K, Fetting J. Prevalence of menopausal symptoms among women with a history of breast cancer and attitudes toward estrogen replacement therapy. J Clin Oncol. 1995;13(11):2737-44.
3. Williams RE, Levine KB, Kalilani L, Lewis J, Clark RV. Menopause-specific questionnaire assessment in US population –based study shows negative impact on health-related quality of life. Maturitas. 2009;62(2):153-9.
4. Islam MR, Gartoulla P, Bell RJ, Fradkin P, Davis SR. Prevalence of menopausal symptoms in Asian midlife women: a systematic review. Climacteric. 2015;18(2):157-76.
5. Gold EB, Colvin A, Avis N, Bromberger J, Greendale GA, Powell L, et al. Longitudinal analysis of the association between vasomotor symptoms and race/ethnicity across the menopausal transition: study of women's health across the nation. Am J Public Health. 2006;96(7):1226-35.
6. Randolph JF Jr, Sowers M, Bondarenko I, Gold EB, Greendale GA, Bromberger JT, et al. The relationship of longitudinal change in reproductive hormones and vasomotor symptoms during the menopausal transition. J Clin Endocrinol Metab. 2005;90(11):6106-12.
7. Soules MR, Sherman S, Parrott E, Rebar R, Santoro N, Utian W, et al. Executive summary: Stages of Reproductive Aging Workshop (STRAW). Fertil Steril. 2001;76(5):874-8.
8. Kronenberg F. Hot flashes: epidemiology and physiology. Ann NY Acad Sci. 1990; 592:52-86.
9. Pennebaker J. The psychology of physical symptoms. New York: Springer-Verlag; 1982.
10. Archer DF, Sturdee DW, Baber R, de Villiers TJ, Pines A, Freedman RR, et al. Menopausal hot flushes and night sweats: where are we now? Climacteric. 2011;14(5):515-28.
11. Freedman RR. Hot flashes: behavioral treatments, mechanisms, and relation to sleep. Am J Med. 2005;118(Suppl 12B):124-30.
12. Freedman RR. Physiology of hot flashes. Am J Hum Biol. 2001;13(4):453-64.
13. Casper RF, Yen SS. Neuroendocrinology of menopausal flushes: an hypothesis of flush mechanism. Clin Endocrinol (Oxf). 1985;22(3):293-312.
14. Rance NE, Dacks PA, Mittelman-Smith MA, Romanovsky AA, Krajewski-Hall SJ. Modulation of body temperature and LH secretion by hypothalamic KNDy (kisspeptin, neurokinin B and dynorphin) neurons: a novel hypothesis on the mechanism of hot flushes. Front Neuroendocrinol 2013;34(3):211-27.
15. Freedman RR, Blacker CM. Estrogen raises the sweating threshold in postmenopausal women with hot flashes. Fertil Steril. 2002;77(3):487-90.
16. Crandall CJ, Zheng Y, Crawfold, SL, Thurston RC, Gold EB, Johnston JM, et al. Presence of vasomotor symptoms is associated with lower bone mineral density: A longitudinal analysis. Menopause. 2009;16(2):239-46.
17. Whiteman MK, Starpoll CA, Benedict LC, Borgest C, Flaws JA. Risk factors for hot flashes in midlife women. J Womens Health. 2003;12(5):459-72.
18. Grodin JM, Siiteri PK, MacDonald PC. Source of estrogen production in postmenopausal women. J Clin Endocrinol Metab. 1973;36(2):207-14.
19. MacDonald PC, Edman CD, Hemsell DL, Porter JC, Siiteri PK. Effect of obesity on conversion of plasma androstenedione to estrone in postmenopausal women with and without endometrial cancer. Am J Obstet Gynecol. 1978;130(4):448-55.
20. Gold EB, Sternfeld B, Kelsey JL, Brown C, Mouton C, Reame N, et al. Relation of demographic and lifestyle factors to symptoms in a multi-racial/ethnic population of women 40-55 years of age. Am J Epidemiol. 2000;152(5):463-73.

21. Whiteman MK, Staropoli CA, Langenberg PW, McCarter RJ, Kjerulff KH, Flaws JA. Smoking, body mass, and hot flashes in midlife women. Obstet Gynecol. 2003;101(2):264-72.
22. Huang AJ, Subak LL, Wing R, West DS, Hernandez AL, Macer J, et al. An intensive behavioral weight loss intervention and hot flushes in women. Arch Intern Med. 2010;170(13):1161-7.
23. Thurston RC, Sower MR, Strendfeld B, Gold EB, Bromberger J, Chang Y, et al. Gains in body fat and vasomotor symptoms reporting over the menopausal transition; the study of women's Health across the nation. Am J Epidemiol. 2009;170(6):766-74.
24. Koo S, Ahn Y, Lim JY, Cho J, Park HY. Obesity associates with vasomotor symptoms in postmenopause but with physical symptoms in perimenopause: a cross-sectional study. BMC Women's Health. 2017; (17):126.
25. David PS, Kling JM, Vegunta S, Faubion SS, Kapoor E, Mara KC, et al. Vasomotor symptoms in women over 60: results from the Data Registry on Experiences of Aging, Menopause, and Sexuality (DREAMS). Menopause. 2018;25(10):1105-9.
26. Borkoles E, Reynolds N, Ski CF, Stojanovska L, Thompson DR, Polman RC. Relationship between type D personality, physical activity behavior and climacteric symptoms. BMC Women's Health. 2015;15:1.
27. Romani WA, Gallicchio L, Flaws JA. The physical association between physical activity and hot flash severity, frequency, and duration in mid-life women. Am J Hum Biol. 2009;21(1):127-9.
28. Smith RL, Flaws JA, Gallichio L. Does quitting smoking decrease the risk of midlife hot flashes? A longitudinal analysis. Maturitus. 2015;82:123-7.
29. Crandall CJ, Manson JE, Hohensee C, Horvath S, Wactawski-Wende J, LeBlanc ES, et al. Association of genetic variation in the tachykinin receptor 3 locus with hot flashes and night sweats in the Women's Health Initiative Study. Menopause. 2017;24(3):252-61.
30. Seivert LL, Flanagan EK. Geographical distribution of hot flash frequencies: considering climatic influences. Am J Phys Anthropol. 2005;128(2):437-43.
31. Avis NE, Crawford SL, Greendale G, Bromberger JT, Everson-Rose SA, Gold EB, et al. Duration of menopausal vasomotor symptoms over the menopause transition. JAMA Intern Med. 2015;175(4):531-9.
32. Thurston RC, Sutton-Tyrrell K, Everson-Rose SA, Hess R, Matthews KA. Hot flashes and subclinical cardiovascular disease: findings from the Study of Women's Health Across the Nation Heart Study. Circulation. 2008;118(12):1234-40.
33. Crandall CJ, Tseng CH, Crawford SL, Thurston RC, Gold EB, Johnston JM, et al. Association of menopausal vasomotor symptoms with increased bone turnover during the menopausal transition. J Bone Miner Res. 2011;26(4):840-9.
34. Dennerstein L, Dudley EC, Hopper JL, Guthrie JR, Burger HG. A prospective population-based study of menopausal symptoms. Obstet Gynecol. 2000;96(3):351-8.
35. Kravitz HM, Janssen I, Santoro N, Bromberger JT, Schocken M, Everson-Rose SA, et al. Relationship of day-to-day reproductive hormone levels to sleep in midlife women. Arch Intern Med. 2005;165(20):2370-6.
36. Stuenkel CA, Davis SR, Gompel A, Lumsden MA, Murad MH, Pinkerton JV, et al. Treatment of symptoms of the menopause: An Endocrine Society Clinical Practice Guideline. J Clin Endocrinol Metab. 2015;100(11):3975-4011.
37. Pinkerton JV, Harvey JA, Pan K, Thompson JR, Ryan KA, Chines AA, et al. Breast effects of bazedoxifene-conjugated estrogens: a randomized controlled trial. Obstet Gynecol. 2013;121(5):959-68.
38. Lobo RA, Pinkerton JV, Gass ML, Dorin MH, Ronkin S, Pickar JH. Evaluation of bazedoxifene/conjugated estrogens for the treatment of menopausal symptoms and effects on metabolic parameters and overall safety profile. Fertil Steril. 2009; 92(3):1025-38.

39. Pinkerton JV, Utian WH, Constantine GD, Olivier S, Pickar JH. Relief of vasomotor symptoms with the tissue-selective estrogen complex containing bazedoxifene/conjugated estrogens: a randomized, controlled trial. Menopause. 2009;16:1116.
40. Wildemeersch D. Potential health benefits of continuous LNG-IUS combined with parenteral ERT for seamless menopausal transition and beyond—a commentary based on clinical experience. Gynecol Endocrinol. 2013;29(6):569-73.
41. Sideras K, Loprinzi CL. Nonhormonal management of hot flashes for women on risk reduction therapy. J Natl Compr Canc Netw. 2010;8(10):1171-9.
42. Loprinzi CL, Kugler JW, Sloan JA, Mailliard JA, LaVasseur BI, Barton DL, et al. Venlafaxine in management of hot flashes in survivors of breast cancer: a randomised controlled trial. Lancet. 2000;356(9247):2059-63.
43. Suvanto-Luukkonen E, Koivunen R, Sundström H, Bloigu R, Karjalainen E, Häivä-Mällinen L, et al. Citalopram and fluoxetine in the treatment of postmenopausal symptoms: a prospective, randomized, 9-month, placebo-controlled, double-blind study. Menopause. 2005;12(1):18-26.
44. Stearns V, Beebe KL, Iyengar M, Dube E. Paroxetine controlled release in the treatment of menopausal hot flashes: a randomized controlled trial. JAMA. 2003;289(21):2827-34.
45. Bordeleau L, Pritchard KI, Loprinzi CL, Ennis M, Jugovic O, Warr D, et al. Multicenter, randomized, cross-over clinical trial of venlafaxine versus gabapentin for the management of hot flashes in breast cancer survivors. J Clin Oncol. 2010;28(35):5147-52.
46. Nelson HD, Vesco KK, Haney E, Fu R, Nedrow A, Miller J, et al. Nonhormonal therapies for menopausal hot flashes: systematic review and meta-analysis. JAMA. 2006;295(17):2057-71.
47. Leon-Ferre RA, Novotny PJ, Faubion SS, Ruddy KJ, Flora D, Dakhil C, et al. Abstract GS6-02: A randomized, double-blind, placebo-controlled trial of oxybutynin (Oxy) for hot flashes (HF): ACCRU study SC-1603. Cancer Res. 2019;79(4):GS6.
48. Skorupskaite K, George JT, Veldhuis JD, Millar RP, Anderson RA. Neurokinin 3 receptor antagonism reveals roles for neurokinin B in the regulation of gonadotropin secretion and hot flashes in postmenopausal women. Neuroendocrinology. 2018;106(2):148-57.
49. Modelska K, Cummings S. Tibolone for postmenopausal women: systematic review of randomized trials. J Clin Endocrinol Metab. 2002;87(1):16-23.
50. Jones SE, Cantrell J, Vukelja S, Pippen J, O'Shaughnessy J, Blum JL, et al. Comparison of menopausal symptoms during the first year of adjuvant therapy with either exemestane or tamoxifen in early breast cancer: report of a Tamoxifen Exemestane Adjuvant Multicenter trial substudy. J Clin Oncol. 2007;25(30):4765-71.
51. McCurry SM, Guthrie KA, Morin CM, Woods NF, Landis CA, Ensrud KE, et al. Telephone-Based cognitive behavioral therapy for insomnia in perimenopausal and postmenopausal women with vasomotor symptoms: A MsFLASH randomized clinical trial. JAMA Intern Med. 2016;176(7):913-20.
52. Janet S Carpenter, MLS Gass, Paulin M Maki. Nonhormonal management of vasomotor symptoms. Menopause. 2015;22(11):1155-72.
53. Nedrow A, Miller J, Walker M, Nygren P, Huffman LH, Nelson HD. Complementary and alternative therapies for the management of menopause-related symptoms: a systematic evidence review. Arch Intern Med. 2006;166(14):1453-65.
54. Carmody JF, Crawford S, Salmoirago-Blotcher E, Leung K, Churchill L, Olendzki N. Mindfulness training for coping with hot flashes: results of a randomized trial. Menopause. 2011;18(6):611-20.
55. Keenan NL, Mark S, Fugh-Berman A, Browne D, Kaczmarczyk J, Hunter C. Severity of menopausal symptoms and use of both conventional and complementary/alternative therapies. Menopause. 2003;10(6):507-15.

56. Deng G, Vickers A, Yeung S, D'Andrea GM, Xiao H, Heerdt AS, et al. Randomized, controlled trial of acupuncture for the treatment of hot flashes in breast cancer patients. J Clin Oncol. 2007;25(35):5584-90.
57. Dodin S, Blanchet C, Marc I, Ernst E, Wu T, Vaillancourt C, et al. Acupuncture for menopausal hot flushes. Cochrane Database Syst Rev. 2013;(7):CD007410.
58. Pruthi S, Qin R, Terstreip SA, Liu H, Loprinzi CL, Shah TR, et al. A phase III, randomized, placebo-controlled, double-blind trial of flaxseed for the treatment of hot flashes: North Central Cancer Treatment Group N08C7. Menopause. 2012; 19(1):48-53.
59. Aiello EJ, Yasui Y, Tworoger SS, Ulrich CM, Irwin ML, Bowen D, et al. Effect of a yearlong, moderate-intensity exercise intervention on the occurrence and severity of menopause symptoms in postmenopausal women. Menopause. 2004;11(4):382-8.
60. Daley A, Stokes-Lampard H, Thomas A, MacArthur C. Exercise for vasomotor menopausal symptoms. Cochrane Database Syst Rev. 2014;(11):CD006108.
61. Lindh-Astrand L, Nedstrand E, Wyon Y, Hammar M. Vasomotor symptoms and quality of life in previously sedentary postmenopausal women randomised to physical activity or estrogen therapy. Maturitas. 2004;48(2):97-105.
62. Chattha R, Raghuram N, Venkatram P, Hongasandra NR. Treating the climacteric symptoms in Indian women with an integrated approach to yoga therapy: a randomized control study. Menopause. 2008;15(5):862-70.
63. Othman AH, Zaky AH. Management of hot flushes in breast cancer survivors: comparison between stellate ganglion block and pregabalin. Pain Med. 2014; 15(3):410-7.

CHAPTER 5

Genitourinary Syndrome of Menopause

▪ INTRODUCTION

Menopause is the permanent cessation of menstruation. It is associated with an arrest of ovarian synthesis of estrogen, progesterone, and dehydroepiandrosterone (DHEA).[1] Loss of steroid hormones, particularly estrogen deficiency, causes physical changes that interfere with normal sexual and genitourinary functioning in a significant number of postmenopausal women.[2] Abundant estrogen receptors are present in vulva, vagina, urethra, and vestibule. Estrogen withdrawal due to menopause causes vulvovaginal atrophy (VVA) or dryness of the vagina and decreased blood supply to the urethra and decreased thickness of submucous plexus of the bladder and the urethra. It may be the problem at any age, but it occurs more frequently in women beyond menopause. VVA is a silent epidemic affecting up to 50–60% of postmenopausal women. In the US two-thirds of postmenopausal women suffer from VVA in their lifetime.[3]

The term genitourinary syndrome of menopause (GSM) is new nomenclature of VVA, which is the collection of signs and symptoms associated with the dryness of vagina, dyspareunia, soreness, dysuria, frequency and urgency of urination, and repeated urinary tract infection. The term GSM provides a broader description of the genitourinary effects of estrogen withdrawal in menopause and thus removes the negative stigma of dryness of vagina for women. GSM rather than VVA is a more accurate and inclusive term that describes multiple changes occurring in external genitalia, pelvic floor tissues, bladder, urethra, vagina and sexual function, and decreased libido caused by hypoestrogenism during the menopausal transition and postmenopause. Women spend more than one third of their lives in the postmenopausal state. Over half of postmenopausal women experience GSM[4] and more than 75% report having an impact on their sexual lives. This VVA is a significant determinant of quality-of-life and sexual well-being for menopausal women.[5] Although, the symptoms are diverse, the prevalence is high,[6] the health and quality-of-life of postmenopausal women are severely affected by GSM and GSM is associated with sexual dysfunction[7] but there is less reporting by women. As 70% of women believe that it is natural during menopause, they have to tolerate this agony, so that they do not turn to the doctor and suffer in silence. Moreover, many women believe that the symptoms will subside over time or attribute them to a natural part of aging. Survey revealed that only 20–25% of women with GSM are seeking medical attention **(Fig. 1)**.[8]

Genitourinary Syndrome of Menopause

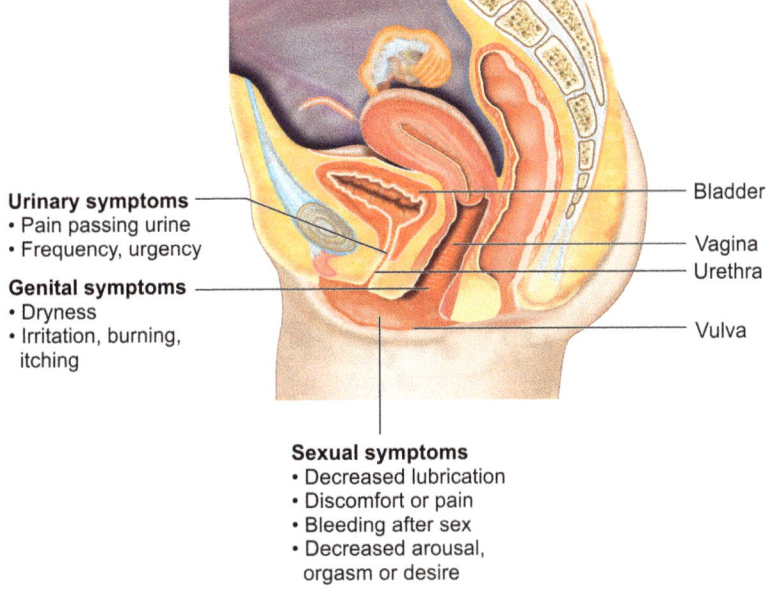

Fig. 1: Anatomy of female genitourinary system.
Source: LECOM (Obs/Gyne, March 3, 2018).

■ SYMPTOMS/SIGNS OF GSM

The GSM focuses on vaginal atrophy, sexual discomfort, and urinary disorders. GSM includes vaginal soreness, vaginal pain, burning, itching in the vagina and mild discharge, overall vaginal discomfort and severe dyspareunia.[9,10] Also GSM/VVA is associated with frequency, urgency, dysuria, nocturnal and urge incontinence. As VVA is inadequate to describe the range of menopausal urogenital symptoms, the International society for the study of Women's Sexual health and the NAMS proposed the term GSM (Genitourinary syndrome of menopause) instead of VVA.[11] GSM has also been adopted as VVA, which includes symptoms and signs such as changes in labia majora or minora, clitoris, vestibules/introitus, vagina, urethra and bladder associated with decreased estrogen, and other sex steroids, so the treatment should be started early to prevent irreversible tissue atrophy.[12,13] GSM/VVA can start in perimenopause, increase during early menopause, and further increase a few years after menopause, with the symptoms ranging from mild to unbearable severity **(Box 1)**.[14]

Anatomical Changes Responsible for the Symptoms

Unlike vasomotor symptoms GSM/VVA does not resolve spontaneously; instead, there is a progressive and cumulative negative effect over the time.[15] Long-term therapy may be necessary to maintain urogenital health, but vaginal application of estrogen has been shown to have the least systemic absorption.[16] Due to aging and changing hormonal milieu, menopause

> **BOX 1:** Genitourinary syndrome of menopause: Clinical symptoms.
> - Vulvovaginal dryness, itching, burning, irritation
> - Vaginal discharge
> - Decreased lubrication or arousal with sexual activity
> - Pain with introital insertion during sexual activity (dyspareunia)
> - Decreased or delayed orgasm
> - Postcoital bleeding
> - Dysuria
> - Urinary frequency or urgency
> - Recurrent urinary tract infections
>
> *Source:* Cleveland Clinic Journal of Medicine, May 2018.

encompasses VVA, urinary, and pelvic manifestations associated with, and further potential etiology. The lack of sex steroid during menopause also causes a decrease in the proportion of superficial cells and an increase in the proportion of immature parabasal cells.[17] GSM or VVA affects half of menopausal women who have severe sexual dysfunction. Vaginal dryness causes severe dyspareunia, which again results in poor arousal, impaired orgasm and consequently, reduced sexual satisfaction. Women with symptoms of VVA or GSM also often have sexual dysfunction,[18] vasomotor symptoms, depression and multiple coexisting conditions, such as osteoporosis and urinary incontinence.[19,20]

Anatomical changes related to GSM include: thinning of the vaginal mucosa, mucosal dryness, elastic and collagen tissue atrophy with reduced blood supply. Menopause results in altered appearance and function of smooth muscle cells, increased density of connective tissue, and fewer blood vessels, a rise in vaginal pH, which is the index of poor vaginal epithelium maturation, indicates estrogen deficiency and results in chronic VVA or GSM.[21,22] There are also changes in vaginal flora associated with the loss of superficial cells, glycogen, and lactobacilli resulting in increased pH and increased potential for vaginal and urinary tract infection and inflammation.[23] Decreased blood supply and less elasticity make the vagina prone to petechiae, injury, and pain **(Fig. 2)**.[24]

Effect of Estrogen Deficiency

Estrogen withdrawal causes thinning, narrowing, shrinking of blood supply, decreased lubrication, and severe dyspareunia again single entity of dyspareunia deteriorates all the domains of female sexual function such as low desire, poor arousal, orgasm, and reduced sexual satisfaction.

In addition, under condition of estrogen deficiency, the balance of the vaginal microbial is disrupted, the pathogenic gram-negative fecal flora and other bacteria prevail in its composition, and instead of acidic the vagina develops alkaline pH, which further causes more deterioration of VVA or GSM **(Fig. 3)**.

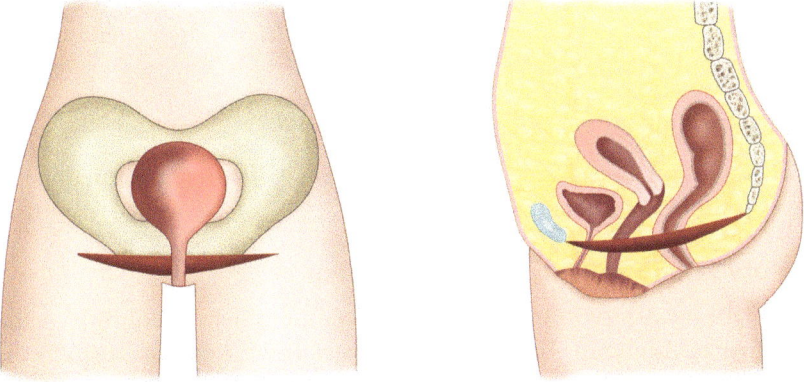

Fig. 2: Impact of menopause on pelvic floor.

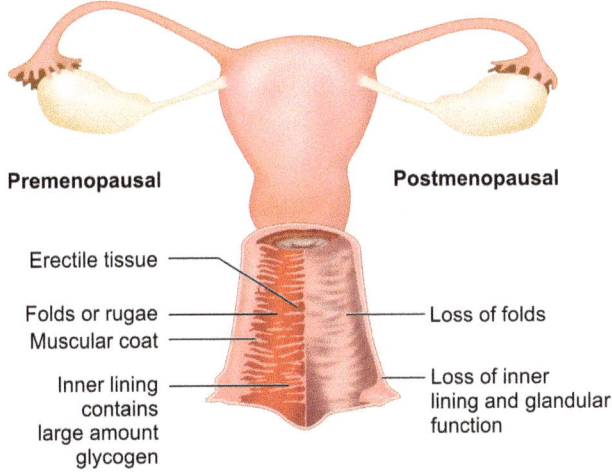

Fig. 3: Changes of vaginal mucosa due to estrogen deficiency.

The effect of these symptoms on quality-of-life often makes it necessary to start treatment immediately, otherwise this condition will become chronic and progressive and devastating.

VVA or GSM brings disharmony in conjugal life; it has significant impact on women's sexuality and quality-of-life.[25] Despite high prevalence and associated burdens, GSM/VVA is often inadequately identified and addressed.[26,27] GSM/VVA is often ignored by women and overlooked by health providers or doctors. Women feel embarrassed to address VVA and this embarrassment appears to be reinforced by perceived lack of interest of the doctors, also doctors do not take into account the impact of GSM/VVA on women's quality-of-life.[28,29]

Although menopausal estrogen deficiency is the leading causes of GSM/VVA, health providers need to exclude other causes of GSM or VVA;

other causes include: smoking cigarette, breastfeeding and puerperium (in younger women), oophorectomy, Sjögren's syndrome, drugs, radiotherapy, infection by bacteria, yeast, and parasite.

■ DIAGNOSIS OF GSM/VVA

It is important to ask questions about GSM whenever postmenopausal woman comes for any check-up.

History Taking and Physical Examination

These are necessary in order to exclude all the other causes of VVA than menopause. Minimum investigations are needed. Women are oblivious about the symptoms even the VIVA (vaginal health; insight, views and attitude) survey showed that the respondents had very little knowledge of vaginal atrophy.[30] Both health care providers (HCPs) and patients find it difficult to discuss vaginal symptoms as a sensitive issue,[27] as evidenced by numerous surveys.[31] Only 36% of HCP in the Revealing Vaginal Effects at Mid Life (REVEAL) survey indicated that they discuss sex-related vaginal pain with their patients.[32] So International Menopause Society (IMS) recommended, that all the Doctors and HCP should be proactive in taking the detail history pointing toward GSM.

Negative Impact on Relationship

The Revive (Real women's views of treatment options for menopausal vaginal changes) survey of 3,046 postmenopausal women with GSM showed that VVA had negative impact on the ability to be intimate 62%, to enjoy sexual intercourse 65%, to be intimate 61%, women's relationship with partner 55%, and sexual spontaneity 54%.[33]

Impact of GSM on Sexuality

Clarifying Vaginal Atrophy's impact on Sex and Relationship (CLOSURE) survey of postmenopausal women in North America, vaginal discomfort was reported to cause participants to avoid intimacy by 58%, to experience loss of libido by 64%, to experience sex-related pain by 64%, and to stop having sex by 30%.[34] The painful ramifications of vaginal atrophy, lead to severe inferiority complex, low self-esteem and depression. Women are oblivious and reluctant to discuss this issue, so empathetic and proactive history of focusing on this particular issue is again very important. Physical examination reveals the atrophic changes of vulva and vagina (**Fig. 4**).

Investigations are done only to exclude the other causes. The maturation index and the pH estimation may be done, but this is not essential. If pH > 5.5 is present in the vagina, it indicates VVA. Routine examination of urine must be checked. Other tests should be carried out on a necessary basis.

Genitourinary Syndrome of Menopause

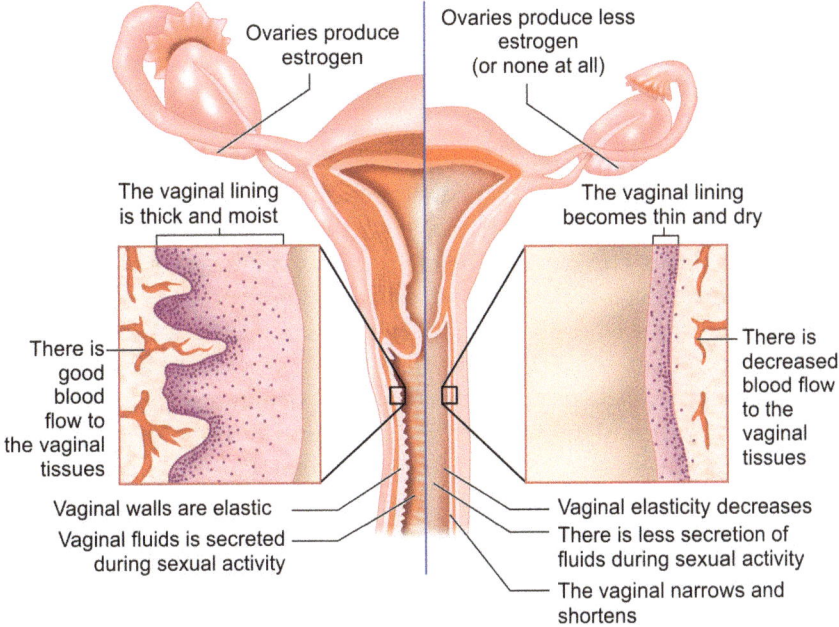

Fig. 4: Physical examination reveals the changes of vagina.
Courtesy: Women's Health.

■ TREATMENT OF GSM/VVA

Treatment depends on the severity of the symptoms of the disease and the preference and expectations of women. The main goal of the treatment is to improve and ameliorate the symptoms of VVA and to restore the anatomical changes to prevent the progression of the disease process. Basically, the treatments include:
- General treatment
- Hormonal treatment
- Nonhormonal therapy.

General Treatment

Maintenance of optimum body weight, regular exercise, yoga, meditation and having optimum nutrition and regular coitus practice, improve GSM to some extent. Women should also be advised to quit smoking and drink too much alcohol. Regular exercise, pelvic floor physiotherapy improves GSM/VVA by increasing the blood flow to the perineum. Positive Attitude of women toward menopause (Swan Study) and awareness causes the mental conditioning of menopausal symptoms. In addition to general treatment, stepwise treatment based on symptoms of severity with both hormonal and nonhormonal options are recommended for women with symptoms that are specially related to sexual activity.[35]

Lubricants and Moisturizers

For mild and moderate VVA, first-line recommendation is lubricants and moisturizers. Regular sex activity is also advised along with lubricants. Moisturizers or lubricants are good alternative to estrogen cream. Women are temporarily relieved by symptoms that ease the dryness of vagina and relieve the painful intercourse. But drawback is that the underlying condition of estrogen deficiency cannot be treated.

Lubricants are administered before sex or as needed to reduce friction, whereas moisturizers are used for 1–3 days with longer effects.[36]

There are three types of lubricants, water-based such as K-Y jelly, silicon-based, and oil-based like Vaseline, petroleum jelly. water-soluble jelly or water-based gel can be used in order to avoid discomfort specifically during sexual activity. These lubricants can be used externally on the labia or clitoris, at the vaginal opening in order to facilitate intromission.[37] Petroleum-based lubricants can be irritating to the vagina, while water-based lubricants may dry the area of application without prolonged activity.[38] Both natural oil- and silicon-based lubricants are not irritating to the vagina but natural oil-based lubricants cannot be used in women with peanut allergies. Silicon-based lubricants are also long-lasting and waterproof.[38] Women should try different products until they find one that meets their needs and to find the one they like best.

Moisturizers provide longer-term relief, rehydrate dry vaginal tissues by changing the fluid content of the vaginal epithelium, absorb and adhere to the epithelium, mimicking vaginal secretions and lowering the pH of the vagina, but no lubricants or moisturizers offer long-term efficacy. Application is simple and convenient, only minority of women (breast cancer survivors) have reported being satisfied with these approaches and had no increased risk of de novo breast cancer like local estrogen therapy (ET).[36,38,39] Lubricants are combinations of protectants and thickening agents in a water base and are temporary measures to relieve vaginal dryness. They must be applied frequently for continuous relief. Lubricants can be helpful early in the course of vaginal atrophy; however, with time, these agents offer little relief and do not restore the integrity of the vagina.

Hormonal Treatment

Considering the cause hypoestrogenism and the pathogenesis of the development of GSM/VVA, the most logical choice for this treatment is ET. Most physician and scientific societies, however, are also looking for other options. Replenishment of estrogen deficiency can be carried out with hormone preparation with systemic and local action. According to latest clinical guidelines, topical estrogen is the preferred drug for GSM or vaginal dryness. Local ET improves the thickness of the vaginal mucosa, reduces pH and increase vaginal maturation index, and improves the signs/symptoms of GSM/VVA (**Fig. 5**).

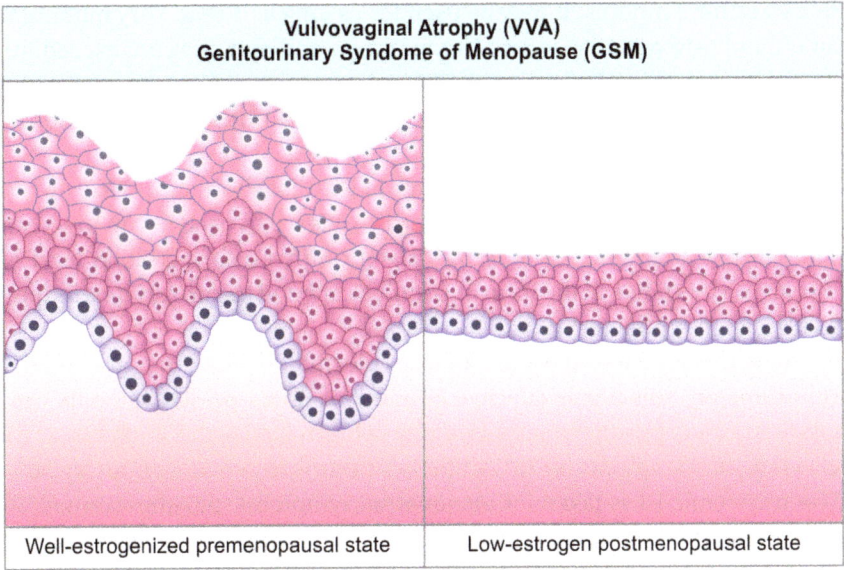

Fig. 5: Histopathological changes of vaginal mucosa.
Courtesy: Adjunct Professor of LECOM, March 3, 2018.

Systemic hormone replacement therapy includes all the estrogen-containing preparation of different formulations. Local estrogen is highly effective in reversing physiological changes associated with GSM/VVA; it fosters vaginal cell growth and maturation, favors lactobacillus colonization, and is preferred in the presence of isolated VVA. The effect of local ET is usually achieved within 1–3 months. Local ET can be administered as vaginal tablets, vaginal cream, or through vaginal ring. The choice of product can be based on clinical experience and patient's preference.[40] It could take weeks for symptoms relief, post-treatment initiation and treatment should continue as long as patients feel discomfort from symptoms.[40] In comparison to cream, tablets have reduced risk of systemic absorption, reduced leakage, and may be better able to deliver a specific dose.[41] Another option-vaginal ring that may be difficult to insert, can be dislodged or may be felt by a partner during sex, if not removed prior to intercourse. All local estrogen alleviates GSM/VVA with similar efficacy.[16] Vaginal ET also has beneficial effects on urinary problems, a meta-analysis of 14 studies showed that ET improved dysuria, urinary urgency, frequency, nocturnal and incontinence.[42] Low-dose ET is preferred to systemic ET, if the goal is to treat the symptoms associated with GSM/VVA.[43] The adverse effect of vaginal estrogen is rare. Women may complain about vaginal irritation, slight vaginal bleeding, but this is rare.

Estrogen local cream is very effective; it is commonly used with estradiol and conjugated equine estrogen. Estradiol is dispensed in the form of tablet vagifem, cream, and ring-estring. Estradiol local cream may be used 50 μg daily; premarin 0.625 mg once daily for 2 weeks and then can be used for twice in a week for 3 months. It may be used for as long as 1 year. Very minimum amount of estrogen is absorbed in the system and that does not exceed the postmenopausal level of estradiol. This amount does not cause endometrial hyperplasia, therefore additional progestins are not recommended during the use of estrogen cream.[44]

These low-dose preparations are safe at least for short term. They do not spur any significant growth of endometrial cells when used for up to 1 year. The estrogen ring and tablet do not significantly boost the blood level of estrogen. The choice of the form of administration of the drug is determined by the patient's preference.

Nevertheless, any postmenopausal bleeding should be evaluated.[35] Unfortunately, this highly effective ET remains under-prescribed, only with less than 10% of postmenopausal women being treated with ET.[45] Systemic ET also reduces symptoms by 75% while local estrogen reduces about 80-90%. When systemic ET is taken for menopausal symptoms, the improvement in well-being with symptoms alleviation may result in improved libido and relief of GSM/VVA.[46] In addition, ET is associated with urinary tract benefits. These include a reduction in the incidence of repeated urinary tract infections and overactive bladder symptoms. Urgencies and stress incontinence, however, do not significantly improve with ET alone.

Testosteron Cream

Existing data provides some support for Testosterone Cream for GSM/VVA as it stimulates vaginal mucosa and improves vaginal dryness by binding the androgen receptor. A woman who suffers from GSM and decreased libido, testosterone is the choice of drug. Intravaginal testosterone administered alone or with vaginal estrogen cream has been shown to improve dyspareunia, sexual desire, lubrication and satisfaction. Beneficial effects are seen three times in a week.[47] But large data is required for routine recommendation.

Vaginal Dehydroepiandrosterone (DHEA)

Dehydroepiandrosterone (Prasterone cream) is a prohormone in the biosynthetic pathways of testosterone and estradiol. It is novel in its conversion into estrogen and testosterone and has undergone robust and formal drug development to confirm its efficacy and safety. This cream better penetrates the vaginal wall. It increases the vaginal wall thickness, elasticity and vascularity of vaginal wall. It improves dyspareunia and libido along with GSM/VVA.[14] It does not stimulate the endometrium.[2] Labrie et al. showed its beneficial effects on VVA and improves dyspareunia and dramatically improves GSM.[29] A study by Barbara Hoffman expressed the high satisfaction of women with DHEA. Daily dose of intravaginal application of DHEA (6.5 mg) has shown favorable effects on vaginal dryness and dyspareunia, but these effects are not sustained when given twice a week and RCTs have not shown benefits of its effect on systemic therapy. In both pivotal trials, treatment with intravaginal Prasterone (DHEA) was associated with reduction in moderate to severe dyspareunia for women with menopause, compared to placebo, (−1.27, 0.40 severity score units over placebo, 46%; $p = 0.003$) and (−1.42, 0.36 severity score units over placebo, 34%; $p \leq 0.0002$) in pivotal trial 1 and 2, respectively.[48] For the daily vaginal use of DHEA, Intrarosa® (prasterone) (6.5 mg) was approved by the FDA for use in the treatment of dyspareunia. Regarding endometrial safety—multicenter, placebo-controlled trial showed atrophy or inactive endometrium, found from histopathology obtained from users of Prasterone with no proliferation or hyperplasia of the endometrium, confirming the lack of stimulatory effect of intravaginal Prasterone.[49] Many postmenopausal women suffering with GSM/VVA identify painful intercourse is the most bothersome symptom. Prasterone can provide a safe, effective, and innovative approach to this common and often debilitating condition.

Nonhormonal Treatment

Ospemifene is a selective estrogen receptor modulator (SERM), used 60 mg/day. It is albeit a systemic nonhormonal therapy, it acts locally as an estrogen. It interacts with intracellular estrogen receptors in the target organs as agonist or antagonist. It has agonist effect on the vaginal epithelium. Its antagonist effect on the endometrium and breast makes it unique and safe; it has no estrogenic effect here. It is the best option when women have contraindication for estrogen, FDA approved Ospemifene for the treatment of moderate to severe dyspareunia caused by GSM/VVA in menopausal women.[2] Beauty of Ospemifene is that it can improve sexual function (desire, arousal, orgasm, lubrication, satisfaction and reduced pain) in postmenopausal women with GSM/ VVA.[50] It is safe and very effective but better to avoid in women at risk of thromboembolism.[26] Ospemifene is a third-generation SERM indicated for treatment of moderate-to-severe symptomatic VVA in postmenopausal women, Ospemifene is administered orally, thus avoiding the inconveniences of local therapy. Ospemifene is the only therapeutic option approved for use in women with VVA. It is well-tolerated for short and long-term use. Endometrium remains atrophic after 12 months meta-analyses have indicated that Ospemifene significantly improves morphological and physiological features of the vaginal mucosa associated with postmenopausal VVA[13] and has a good safety profile. The analyses examined six randomized controlled trials (RCTs) of Ospemifene *versus* placebo involving 2086 women, who were followed for up to 52 weeks. Changes observed in vaginal pH, parabasal cells, superficial cells, and dyspareunia after weeks' treatment were significantly in favor of Ospemifene over placebo (all $p < 0.0001$).[13] No differences were observed between Ospemifene and placebo at 12 or 52 weeks in incidences of headaches, deep vein thrombosis, coronary heart disease, cardiovascular events, number of treatment discontinuations due to adverse events, or serious adverse events.[51] In addition, Ospemifene reduces the bone turnovers. A positive cascade effect on other domains of sexual function has been documented. Lasofoxifene is a new third generation SERM. It also binds both receptors and it shows same efficacy, but is not yet approved by the FDA **(Table 1)**.

Laser Therapy

Laser therapy is the newer option of treatment for GSM/VVA. There are very few options available, local ET seems to be superior to others but still not very much effective compared to placebo. Kozma et al. confidently concluded from their study that fractional CO_2 laser is an effective and safe treatment of GSM-associated symptoms.[52] In addition, the REVIVE study suggests that women are concerned about long-term use and safety of vaginal ET.[53] In this context, laser therapy is very promising. Laser technology delivers fractional CO_2 and nonablative photo thermal Er:YAG to the vaginal wall. Both the groups are simple, faster, and painless. They differ in wavelength, water absorption, and tissue penetration. Both activate dominant fibroblasts to increase collagen tissue, proteoglycans, and hyaluronic acid inside the vagina. Therefore water is retained in vagina and blood supply to the vaginal mucosa becomes normal. Laser therapy replenishes glycogen in the vaginal mucosa and restores pH balance of mucosa and therefore improves the symptoms of atrophy and improves sexuality.[30] The Salvatore study showed that 85% of women regained sexuality within 12 weeks of laser therapy.[33] Long-term data have shown that improvement of vaginal health may continue up to 24 months after fractional CO_2 and 80% of women have decided to start a new treatment cycle of laser applications. Laser therapy has demonstrated high satisfaction among patients and HCPs. Menopausal hormone therapy (MHT) can provide quick and long-term relief while urinary symptoms often require additional effective therapy.[54] A recent systemic review and meta-analysis of 14 observational studies found that all symptoms of GSM/VVA and urinary incontinence significantly decreased and marked improvement in sexual function[55] with laser treatment **(Fig. 6)**.

Women need to choose, considering the benefits and risks associated with each strategy. A systematic review and meta-analysis reported that, despite the lack of well-designed controlled studies, laser intervention appears to be safe and potentially effective nonpharmacological intervention for GSM/VVA. It induces a significant improvement in vaginal health.[56]

Newer Generation of Laser

Erbium laser is nonablative photo thermal therapy that is very effective, but ACOG has not yet recommended its use. Cardozo et al. conducted the first randomized, single blind, multicenter study of both laser types, which proved

TABLE 1: Nonhormonal therapy for VVA.

Treatment type	Specific therapy	Typical use	Notes
Education	Educate regarding potential vulvar and vaginal changes associated with menopause or other low estrogen state; offer therapy as indicated		Education should be offered to women regardless of partner status; regular painless sexual activity or vaginal stimulation can help maintain sexual function
Counseling and sex therapy	Cognitive behavioral therapy; mindfulness exercises		Counseling or sex therapy with a qualified counselor/therapist may be useful for women with dyspareunia or relationship discord. AASECT.org
Lubricants	Water-based Silicone-based Oil-based	Used as needed for sexual activity	Used to increase comfort and pleasure; avoid potential irritants (e.g., glycerin, parabens, propylene glycol); can be used with other therapies (hormone and nonhormone)
Moisturizers		Used daily or every few days on a regular basis independent of sexual play to maintain vulvar and vaginal moisture	Mimics normal vaginal secretions; does not restore or reverse cellular/pH changes of GSM; can be used with other therapies (hormone and nonhormone)
Self-stimulators/ Vibrators	May be a variety of materials (e.g., latex, nonlatex, silicone, hard plastic)	Can be used as needed during sexual play, alone, or with partner	Gently stimulates vulvar and vaginal tissues; may facilitate natural lubrication; may help maintain function
Dilators	May be a variety of materials (e.g., plastic, silicone, glass)	Ideal duration or frequency of use is unknown	Stretches vaginal tissues
Pelvic floor physical therapy	Examples: education on kinesthetic awareness; pelvic floor muscle relaxation; manual therapies; biofeedback	Used as needed for nonrelaxing pelvic floor muscle dysfunction	Identify a physical therapist who specializes in pelvic floor disorders www.womenshealthapta.org/

(AASECT: American Association of Sexuality Educators, Counselors, and Therapists; GSM: genitourinary syndrome of menopause)
Source: Adapted from Faubion S, et al.

safety and efficacy of laser treatment for GSM/VVA. Therefore, it can be said that vaginal laser has been shown to restore the virginal's physiology and effectively treat GSM/VVA.[57]

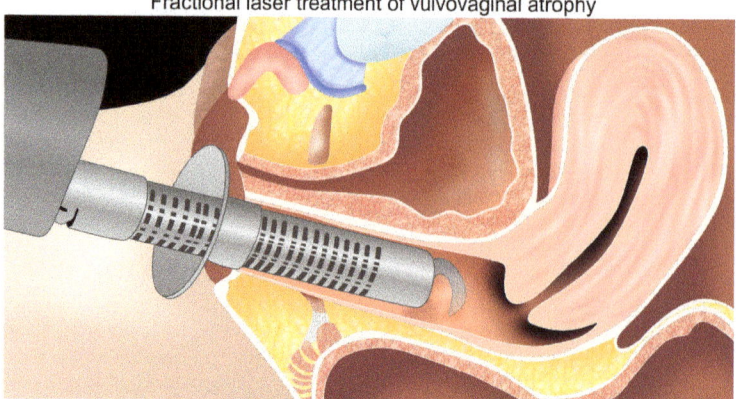

Fig. 6: Technique of laser administration.

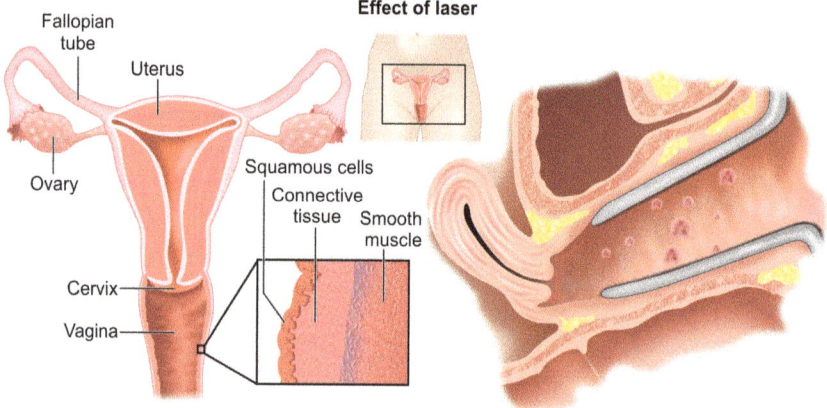

Fig. 7: Improvement of vaginal mucosa.

Nonhormonal therapy: Antidepressant, Gabapentin, Serotonin reuptake inhibitors, Nor-epinephrine reuptake inhibitors, usually has role to diminish the vasomotor symptoms, but their role for VVA or GSM is not that good.

Plants like Soya (isoflavin), black cohosh, Red clover, Chinese herbs like tofu, mace and flaxseed are used to relieve other menopausal symptoms. It is unlikely that GSM/VVA will respond to these drugs. They are not yet evidenced based **(Fig. 7)**.

Probiotics

Oral vitamin D and vaginal vitamin E increases moisture of vagina but the efficacy data are limited. Oral and vaginal probiotics are supposed to alter microbial in favor of GSM/VVA but comprehensive trials are needed for validation.[58]

Pelvic Physical Therapy

Women who do not respond to conventional therapies or hormones are contraindicated with physical therapy may be chosen. Vaginal dilators are the component of physical therapy that may be used in case of vaginal stenosis or shortening of vagina. Some data suggest that dilators improve vaginal function,[59] but are unable to restore the hypoestrogenic effect in vagina.

G-Shot; rejuvenate the orgasm system by stimulating stem cell, found in tissue of vagina and clitoris. Plasma-rich protein (PRP), Botox are being used, many women may get good respond but these treatments for GSM or VVA are not yet evidence based.

■ KEY MESSAGES

- Genitourinary syndrome of menopause or VVA may need not to be an inevitable consequence of menopause. Due to reduced estrogen and sex hormone women suffer from vaginal dryness, burning irritation, dyspareunia, and repeated urinary tract infection.
- Proper diagnosis and intervention with hormone therapy may ameliorate these symptoms and prevent chronic progression.
- A careful history, physical examination is essential in ruling out other vulvovaginal conditions and determining the range and severity of GSM.
- Women may remain silent, although few women may report it, but that is only the tip of the iceberg. Health providers need to break the iceberg of silence and offer full information about different options of treatments of VVA or GSM.
- Local hormone therapy is very effective in moderate to severe degree of GSM. Recurrent urinary tract infection improves with local ET. This therapy may be continued for up to 1 year, Progesterone supplementation is not needed. Laser therapy is very promising treatment.
- All women have right to lead a quality life, so health provider should not only have wide knowledge about the management of GSM/VVA, but they need to be very kind and should have empathy.
- Shared decision-making between physician and patients is the key of success to treat GSM/VVA, early intervention prevent the progression of disease process.

■ REFERENCES

1. Labrie F, Belanger A, Pelletier G, Martel C, Archer DF, Utian WH. Science of intracrinology in postmenopausal women. Menopause. 2017;24:702-12.
2. Davis SR, Davison SL, Donath S, Bell RJ. Circulating androgen levels and self-reported sexual function in women. JAMA. 2005;294:91-6.
3. Krychman M, Graham S, Bernick B, Mirkin S, Kingsburg SA. The women's EMPOWER survey; women's knowledge and awareness of treatment options for vulvar and vaginal atrophy remains inadequate. J Sex Med. 2017;14;425-33.
4. Erekson EA, Li FY, Martin DK, Fried TR. Vulvovaginal symptoms prevalence in postmenopausal women and relationship to other menopausal symptoms and pelvic floor disorders. Menopause. 2016;23:363-75.
5. Nappi RE, Palacios S. Impact of vulvovaginal atrophy on sexual health and quality of life at postmenopause. Climacteric. 2014;17:3-9.
6. Calleja-Agius J, Brincat MP. Urogenital atrophy. Climacteric. 2009;12:279-85.

7. Lara LA, Useche B, Ferriani RA, Reis RM, de Sá MF, de Freitas MM, et al. The effects of hyopoestrogenism on the vaginal wall: Interference with the normal sexual response. J Sex Med. 2009;6:30-9.
8. Wysoki S, Kingsberg S, Krychman M. Management of vaginal atrophy: Implications from the REVIVE Survey. Clin Med Insights Reprod Health. 2014;8:23-30.
9. Santoro N, Komi J. Prevalence and impact of vaginal symptoms among postmenopausal women. J Sex Med. 2009;6:2133-42.
10. Santoro N, Sherman S. New interventions for menopausal symptoms. Bethesda MD: National institute of Health, UD Department of Health and Human Services; 2006.
11. Portman DJ, Gass ML, Vulvovaginal Atrophy Terminology Consensus Conference Panel. Genitourinary Syndrome of menopause: New terminology for vulvovaginal atrophy from The International Society for the Study of Women' Sexual Health and The North American Menopause Society. Climacteric. 2014;17;557-63.
12. Shaprio M. What should guide our patient management of vulvovaginal atrophy? Climacteric. 2019;22(1): 38-43.
13. Baber RJ, Panay N, Fenton A; IMS Writing Group. 2016 IMS Recommendation on women's midlife health and menopause hormone therapy. Climacteric. 2016;19;109-50.
14. Freedman MA. Perceptions of dyspareunia in postmenopausal women with vulvar and vaginal atrophy: findings from the REVIVE survey. Womens Health (Lond Engl). 2014;10:445-54.
15. Barton DL, Shuster LT, Dockter T, Atherton PJ, Thielen J, Birrell SN, et al. Systemic and local effects of vaginal dehydroepiandrosterone (DHEA): NCCTG N10C1 (Alliance). Support Care Cancer. 2018;26:1335-43.
16. Lethaby A, Ayeleke R, Roberts H. Local estrogen for vaginal atrophy in postmenopausal women. Cochrane Database Syst Rev. 2016;8:CD00150.
17. Meisels A. The menopause: a cytohormonal study. Acta Cytol. 1966;10:59-5.
18. Nappi RE, Cucinella L, Martella S. Female sexual dysfunction (FSD); prevalence and impact on quality of life. Maturitas. 2016;94:87-91.
19. Worsley R, Bell RJ, Gartoulla P, Davis SR. Prevalence and predictors of low sexual desire, sexuality related personal distress and hypoactive sexual desire dysfunction in a community based sample of midlife women. J Sex Med. 2007;14:675-86.
20. Sidi H, Puteh SE, Abdullah N, Midin M. The prevalence of sexual dysfunction and potential risk factors that may impair sexual function in Malaysian women. J Sex Med. 2007;4:311-21.
21. Johnston S. Urological concerns. J Obstet Gynecol Can. 2006;28:533-42.
22. North American Menopause Society. The role of local vaginal estrogen for the treatment of vaginal atrophy in postmenopausal women. 2007 position statement of the North American Society. Menopause. 2007;14:355-69.
23. Willhite LA, O'Connell MB. Urogenital atrophy: Prevention and treatment. Pharmacotherapy. 2001;21:464-80.
24. Mac Bride MB, Rhodes DJ, Shuster LT. Vulvovaginal atrophy. Mayo Clin Proc. 2010;85:87-9.
25. Nappi RE, Lachowsky M. Menopause and sexuality; prevalence of symptoms and impact on quality of life. Maturitas. 2009;63;138-41.
26. Palma F, Volpe P, Villa P, Cagnacci A; Writing Group of the AGATA STUDY. Vaginal atrophy of women in postmenopause. Results from multicentric observational study: The AGATA study. Maturitas. 2016;83:40-4.
27. Kingsberg SA, Wysocki S, Magnus L. Vulvar and vaginal atrophy in postmenoausal women; findings from REVIVE (REal Women's VIews of Treatment Options for Menopausal Vaginal ChangEs) survey. J Sex Med. 2013;10:1790-9.
28. Simon JA, Komi J. Postmenopausal women's attitude: Vulvovaginal atrophy and its symptoms (NAMS Abstract LB-10). Menopause. 2007;14:1107.

29. Goldstein I. Recognizing and treating urogenital atrophy in postmenopausal women. J Women's Health (Larchmt). 2010;19:425-32.
30. Nappi RE, de Melo NR, Martino M, Celis-Gonzaliz C, Villaseca P, Röhrich S, et al. Vaginal Health: Insights, Views & Attitudes (VIVA-LATAM): Results from a survey in Latin America. Climacteric. 2018;21(4):397-403.
31. Kingsberg SA, Krychman M, Graham S, Bernick B, Mirkin S. The women's EMPOWER survey: Identifying women's perceptions on vulvar and vaginal atrophy and its treatment. J Sex Med. 2017;14:413-24.
32. Kingsberg SA, Krychman ML. Resistance and barriers to local estrogen therapy in women with atrophic vaginitis. J Sex Med. 2013;10:1567-74.
33. Chua Y, Lympaphayom KK, Cheng B, Ho CM, Sumapradja K, Altomare C, et al. Genitourinary syndrome of menopause in five Asian countries; results from the Pan Asian REVIVE survey. Climacteric. 2017;20:73.
34. Simon JA, Nappi RE, Kingsberg SA, Maamari R, Brown V. Clarifying vaginal atrophy's impact on sex and relationship (CLOSER) survey; emotional and physical impact of vaginal discomfort on North America postmenopausal women their partners. Menopause. 2014;21:137-42.
35. The North American Menopause Society. Management of symptomatic vulvovaginal atrophy: 2013 position statement of The North American Menopause Society. Menopause. 2013;20:888-902.
36. Kingsberg S, Wysocki S, Magnus L, Krychman ML. Vulvar and vaginal atrophy in postmenopausal women: findings from the REVIVE (REal Women's VIews of Treatment Options for Menopausal Vaginal ChangEs) survey. J Sex Med. 2013;10:1790-9.
37. Kingsberg SA, Kellogg S, Krychman M. Treating dyspareunia caused by vaginal atrophy: a review of treatment options using vaginal estrogen therapy. Int J Women's Health. 2009;1:105-11.
38. Hutcherson HY, Kingsberg SA, Krychman ML, Schwartz PJ, Leiblum SR, Rosen RC, et al. A positive approach to female sexual health: a summary report. Female Patient. 2009;(Suppl April): 1-4.
39. Crandall CJ, Hovey KM, Andrews CA, Chlebowski RT, Stefanick ML, Lane DS, et al. Breast cancer, endometrial cancer, and cardiovascular events in participants who used vaginal estrogen in the Women's health initiative observational study. Menopause. 2018;25:11-20.
40. The North American Menopause Society. The role of local vaginal estrogen for treatment of vaginal atrophy in postmenopausal women: 2007 position statement of The North American Menopause Society. Menopause. 2007;14:357-69.
41. Bachmann G, Lobo RA, Gut R, Nachtigall L, Notelovitz M. Efficacy of low-dose estradiol vaginal tablets in the treatment of atrophic vaginitis: a randomized controlled trial. Obstet Gynecol. 2008;111:67-76.
42. Rahn DD, Carberry C, Sanses TV. Vaginal estrogen for genitourinary syndrome of menopause. Obstet Gynecol. 2014;124:1147-56.
43. Archer DF. Efficacy and tolerability of local estrogen therapy for urogenital atrophy. Menopause. 2010;17:194-203.
44. Lullia Naumova, Camil Castelo Branco. Current treatment ooption of postmenopausal vaginal atrophy. Int J Women's Health. 2018;10:387-395.
45. Zeleke BM, Bell RJ, Billah B, Davis SR. Vasomotor and sexual symptoms in older Australian women: A cross-sectional study. Fertil Steril. 2016;105:149-55.e1.
46. Santoro N, Worsley R, Miller KK, Parish SJ, Davis SR. Role of estrogens and estrogen-like compounds in female sexual function and dysfunction. J Sex Med. 2016;13:305-16.
47. Fernandes T, Costa-Pavia LH, Pinto-Neto AM. Efficacy of vaginallt applied estrogen, testosterone or polyacryle acid on sexual function in postmenopausal women: A Randomized controlled acid trial. J Sex Med. 2014;11:1262-7.

48. Labrie F, Archer DF, Kolitun W, Vachon A, Young D, Frenette L, et al. Efficacy of intra vaginal dehydroepiandrosterone (DHEA) on moderate to severe dyspareunia and vaginal dryness, symptoms of vulvovaginal atrophy, and of the genitourinary syndrome of menopause. Menopause. 2016;23:243-56.
49. Simio JA, Goldstein I, Kim NN, Davis SR, Kellogg-Spadt S, Lowenstein L, et al. The role of androgen in the treatment of genitourinary syndrome of menopause (GSM); International society for study of women's Sexual health, expert consensus panel review. Menopause. 2018;25;837-47.
50. Constantine G, Graham S, Portman DJ, Rosen RC, Kingsberg SA. Female sexual function improved with ospemifene in postmenopausal women with vulvar and vaginal atrophy: Results of a randomized, placebo-controlled trial. Climacteric. 2015;18:226-32.
51. Di Donato V, Schiavi MC, Iacobelli V, D'oria O, Kontopantelis E, Simoncini T, et al. Ospemifene for the treatment of vulvar and vaginal atrophy: a meta-analysis of randomized trials. Part II: evaluation of tolerability and safety. Maturitas. 2019;121: 93-100.
52. Kozma B, Póka R, Sipos A, Ács N, Takács P. A hüvelyi CO_2-lézer-kezelés rövid távú hatásai a menopausalis genitourinalis szindróma tüneteire [Short-term efficacy of vaginal CO_2 laser therapy as a treatment modality for genitourinary syndrome of menopause]. Orv Hetil. 2019;160:(41):1617-22.
53. Nappi RE, Palacios S, Panay N, Particco M, Krychman ML. Vulvar and vaginal atrophy in four European countries: Evidence from the European REVIVE survey. Climacteric. 2016;19:188-97.
54. Giarenis I, Cardozo L. Managing urinary incontinence: Why works? Climacteric. 2014; 17 (Suppl 2):26-33.
55. Salvatore S, Nappi RE, Parma M, Chionna R, Lagona F, Zerbinati N, et al. Sexual function after fractional microablative CO_2 laser in women with vulvovaginal atrophy. Climacteric. 2015;18:219-25.
56. Salvator S, Nappi RE, Zerbinati N, Calligaro A, Ferrero S, Origoni M, et al. A 12 week treatment with fractional CO_2 laser for vulvo-vaginal atrophy: A pilot study. Climacteric 2014;17:363-9.
57. Pitsouni E, Grigoriadis T, Falagas ME, Salvatore S, Athanasiou S. Laser therapy for genitourinary syndrome of menopause. A systematic review and meta-analysis. Maturitas. 2017;103:78-88.
58. Muhleisen AL, Herbst-Kralovertz MM. Menopause and the vaginal microbiome. Maturitas. 2016;91:422.
59. Carter J, Goldfrank D, Schover LR. Simple strategies for vaginal health promotion in cancer survivors. J Sex Med. 2011;8;549.

6 Osteoporosis, Bone Health, and Menopause

CHAPTER

■ INTRODUCTION

The age of menopause (51 years) has not changed but life expectancy of women has increased significantly throughout the world. With the average lifespan extended to 70 ± 3 years for women in Bangladesh, most women will spend more than one-third of their lifetime beyond the menopause and may live with consequences of osteoporosis and cardiovascular risks.

Though health concerns of aging women are weight gain, genitourinary syndrome of menopause (GSM), vasomotor symptoms, increased cardiovascular health risks, brain aging with impaired cognition, and disorder of sexual health, osteoporosis is one of the major public health issues because fracture due to osteoporosis is the principal cause of disability and death of elderly women. Menopause leads to bone loss because decreases in estrogen production increase bone resorption and decrease calcium absorption. Annual decrease in bone mass of 3–5% per year frequently occurs in the first years of menopause, but the decrease is typically <1% per year after age of 65 years. Postmenopause status has been associated with increased risk of osteoporosis and fracture. It is estimated that prevalence of osteoporosis is one-third in people of age 50–60 years and 50% or more for over 80 years. By 2050, the global osteoporosis sufferers will reach 6 million (including both males and females), three-fourths of whom will reside in developing countries.[1] One out of three women will experience an osteoporosis-related fracture after menopause, accordingly the lifetime risk of fracture for women at 60 years is 44%, nearly double of the man of the same age.[2] Osteoporosis is the most important risk factor for fall and fracture, which leads to loss of morbidities, autonomy, a reduction of quality life, and development of complications such as pneumonia or thromboembolic diseases which pose considerable health risks and economic burden to public health as, e.g. during the 1st year after fracture, 20–30% of patients died, with the cost amounting to about USD 21,000.[3] Osteoporosis has huge economic burden for the family for the society in our country too. Therefore, osteoporosis is a public health problem, and it needs special attention.

■ DEFINITION AND EPIDEMIOLOGY OF OSTEOPOROSIS

Osteoporosis is defined as a systemic skeletal disease characterized by low bone mass and micro-architectural deterioration of bone tissue leading to enhanced bone fragility and a consequent increase in fracture risk (*NICE clinical guidelines 2012).* Osteoporosis is a disease characterized by low bone mass and disruption of bone architecture, resulting in compromised bone strength and increased fracture risk. Osteoporosis is also considered a silent disease, as there are commonly no symptoms until the first fracture occurs.

Osteoporosis results in significant bone mass loss that decreases bone density and increases the fracture risk. Osteoporotic fracture burden is increasing all over the world. About half of the women aged 50 years and older will have an osteoporosis-related fracture in their lifetime. Alarming fact is 1 in 3 women and 1 out of 5 men >50 years suffer from osteoporosis. It affects 200 million women worldwide (*IOF facts and statistics, 2016*).

Incidence of osteoporotic disability is more than cancers in all over the world. About 50% of all osteoporosis hip fractures will occur by 2050 (IOF) but irony is, osteoporosis is greatly underdiagnosed and undertreated.

Bone is a living tissue with a protein matrix that becomes strong with mineralization (calcium, magnesium, and phosphate). Bone tissues renew/renovate through remodeling process across the lifespan, the overall lifecycle of bone health goal is to build a large, well-mineralized, and strong skeleton or bone mass [bone mineral density (BMD)], so that in future, age-related normal losses would not cause osteoporosis.

The achievement of peak bone mass is important to bone health and plays a vital part in preventing osteoporosis and subsequent fractures in later years. It is reported that hip fractures could be reduced by 30% with an increase in peak bone mass of 10%. Peak BMD is the densest and strongest bone we ever achieve. For women, peak total hip and femoral neck BMD accrue during ages 16–19 years;[4] lumbar spine peak BMD accrue during ages 30–40 years.[5] Many variables are associated with higher peak BMD. These include genetics, gender, ethnicity, region of bones, exercise, exposure to light, and diet.[6] Maintaining adequate calcium intake during childhood is necessary for the development of a maximal peak bone mass. Increasing peak bone mass may be an important way to reduce the risk of osteoporosis in later adulthood.[7] The primary surrogates used are optimization of calcium balance or achievement of greater bone mass in children with increased calcium intake.[8] Bone remodeling process is very important as it maintains the bone mass density. This process is regulated and influenced by several hormones, including parathyroid hormone, calcitonin, 1,25(OH)-vitamin D3, and estrogen. The overall peak BMD is achieved by the age of 30 years.[9]

The SWAN study showed that there is little if any change in BMD in midlife pre- or early perimenopausal women. BMD loss increases substantially in the late menopause and remains rapid in the first few postmenopausal years. During the menopausal transition period, the average reduction in BMD is about 10%. Women lose 50% trabecular bone and 30% cortical bone during course of their life but about half of which is lost during 10 years of

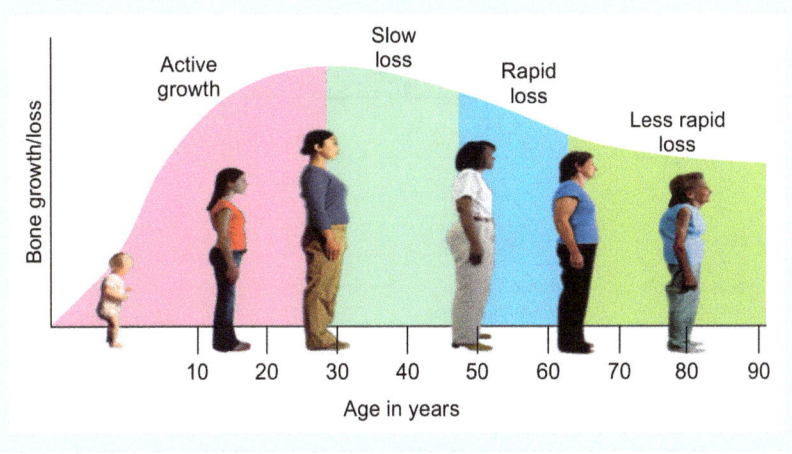

Fig. 1: Bone loss along the age.

menopause.[10] Rapid bone loss due to menopause-related estrogen deficiency eventually causes 40% fracture of all menopause women.[11] Approximately half of the women are losing bone even more rapidly, perhaps as much as 50% in 1st 6-8 years after menopause,[12] those women need to be identified. Bone loss accelerates after the cessation of menstruation at various stages of menopause transition.[13,14] The rate of menopausal bone loss is 1.8-2.3% in spine and 1-1.4% in the hip, the average woman's BMD would decline 7-10% in spine and 5-7% in hip and increase the fracture rate 50-100% higher.[15] Hip fractures are common in osteoporosis, affecting up to 15% women by the age of 80 years.[16] The risk for most fractures is inversely proportional to bone density.[17]

Figure 1 suggests that bone loss is pronounced after the age of 50 years, so healthcare providers should consider screening for osteoporosis when women enter the late stages of the menopause transition, particularly if they have relatively low body weight and risk factors of fractures.

Why menopause has adverse effects on bone health? Adult bone is renovated through two phases, one is unidirectional process of initial removal of old bone called resorption; later it is followed by replacement with new osteoid (bone matrix). Finally mineralization of bone matrix is accomplished. Estrogen is antiresorptive agent. It acts on bone through the estrogen receptors and it helps in:
- Lowering the sensitivity of bone mass to parathyroid hormone, thus reducing bone resorption
- Increasing the production of calcitonin, thus inhibiting bone resorption
- Accelerating calcium absorption by the intestine
- Reducing the calcium excretion from the kidney.

Estrogen, progesterone, and testosterone stimulate bone formation, but cortisol, at high level, enhances bone resorption.

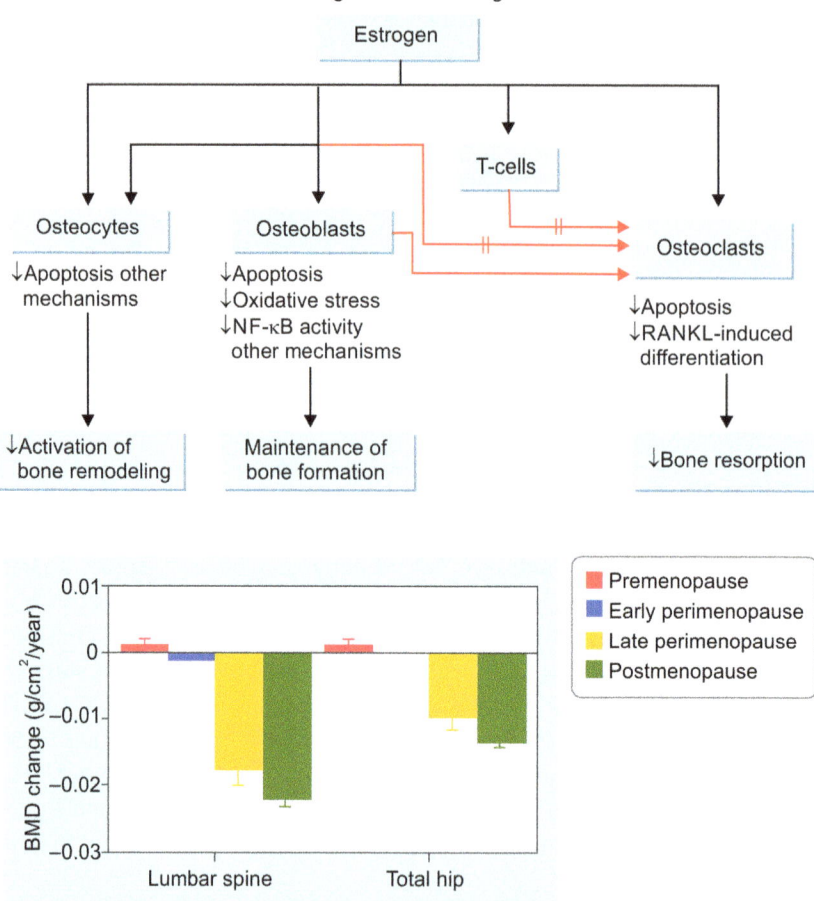

Flowchart 1: Estrogen is the blessing for bone health.

Fig. 2: Rate of bone mineral density (BMD) around menopause.

Therefore, estrogen-deficient state of menopause represents a crucial period in the changes of bone mass density. Estrogen deficiency causes a bone remodeling imbalance with greater increase in the level of osteoclast-mediated bone resorption than osteoblast-mediated bone formation leading to accelerated bone loss and alteration in the microarchitecture of bone **(Flowchart 1)**.

Age after menopause is an important determinant of the rates of bone mass loss.

Along with menopause status **(Fig. 2)**, body size or weight is a major determinant of postmenopausal bone loss and numerous studies have shown that, after menopause, a greater BMD and lower rate of bone loss is seen in overweight and obese women as compared to normal weight women.[18] Study showed that rate of hipbone loss was 50% slower among women who gained weight, even after adjusting their baseline BMD and body

weight.[19] International Society for Clinical Densitometry (ISCD) provides the following *risk factors* for osteoporosis:
- Low calcium intake, anticonvulsants, thin build, ethanol intake hypogonadism, previous fracture, thyroid excess, and race (white, Asian).
- Other relative risk factors with osteoporosis are prolong use of steroids, inactivity or sedentary work, smoking, and delayed menarche.

Secondary causes of osteoporosis are gastrostomy, inflammatory bowel disease, celiac disease, intestinal bypass surgery, primary biliary cirrhosis, and pancreatic insufficiency.

Others are immobilization, renal cause, AIDS/HIV, organ transplantation, chronic obstructive pulmonary disease, anorexia, malignancy, bone marrow-based disorders, hemolytic anemia, multiple myeloma, hemoglobinopathies, myelo and lymphoproliferative, skeletal metastases, Gaucher disease and mastocytosis, inflammatory disorders, rheumatoid arthritis (RA), systemic lupus erythematosus, ankylosing spondylitis, endocrine disorder para/thyroid disease, and diabetes.

■ HOW TO DIAGNOSE OSTEOPOROSIS?

The initial evaluation includes a detailed history taking to assess "clinical risk factors" for bone loss or other morbidities that contribute fracture. Osteoporosis is often called a "silent disease" because initially bone loss occurs without symptoms. Women may not know that they have osteoporosis until their bones become so weak that a sudden strain, bump, or fall causes a fracture or a vertebra to collapse. Collapsed vertebrae may initially be felt or seen in the form of severe back pain, loss of height, or spinal deformities such as stooped posture.

Or many women may complain of chronic back pain.

Physical examination and some basic laboratory tests are necessary for diagnosis. But most important part of history is to find out if there are any risk factors present or not.

Clinical risk factors that contribute to bone loss are advanced age, smoking, excessive alcohol consumption, sedentary habit, previous history of fracture, own fragility fracture, ingestion of steroid, and low body weight. History of previous fracture, especially the fragility fracture, is very important and it is an independent risk factor. Fragility fractures means fractures result from mechanical forces that would not ordinarily result in fracture.

Majority of postmenopausal women with osteoporosis remain asymptomatic or do not show any signs until there is a fracture. But women might complain of persistent unexplained back pain, bone pain, body pain, backache, etc. Loss of height can be the first symptoms of vertebral fracture due to osteoporosis. Physical inactivity and poor nutrition should be addressed. Height and weight need to be measured. The severity of the fracture can be assessed by measuring the extent of vertebral height

TABLE 1: T-score dual-energy X-ray absorptiometry.	
Normal	≥−1
Osteopenia	<−1 and >−2.5
Osteoporosis	≤−2.5
Severe osteoporosis	≤−2.5 with fracture

Source: NICE clinical guideline with WHO, 2012.

reduction by its morphological changes, and by differentiating the fracture from nonfracture deformities. Grades are assigned to each vertebra based on the degree of height reduction.

This patient needs evaluation for other conditions that contribute to bone loss. Early diagnosis and quantification of bone loss and fracture risk are important because of the viability of therapies that can slow or even reverse the progression of osteoporosis.

Bone loss can be measured by measuring the bone mass density. WHO has defined diagnostic threshold for low bone mass and osteoporosis based upon BMD measurement compared with young adult population (T-score). Bone densitometry [dual-energy X-ray absorptiometry (DXA)] is to be done for measurement for BMD. FRAX® (FRAX gives probability of risk of fracture within 10 years). Osteopenia and high FRAX together reflect the risk of major osteoporotic fracture is ≥20% or probability of hip fracture ≥3% within 10 years of time.[20] A clinical diagnosis of osteoporosis may be made in the presence of a fragility fracture, particularly at the spine, hip, wrist, humerus, rib, and pelvis without measurement of BMD. In the absence of fragility fracture, BMD assessment by DEXA is the gold standard to diagnose osteoporosis according to WHO **(Table 1)**.[21] BMD is a strong predictor of fracture risk, majority of fractures occur in women in osteopenia range.

T-score

The WHO established a classification of BMD according to standard deviation (SD) difference between a patient's BMD and that of a young adult reference population (T-score).[22]

If bones are stronger than the average adult, woman's bone mass may be +1 or +2 SD indicating that her bones have a mass 10–20% above that of the average 30-year-old. If bones are less dense than the average adult, woman's standard deviation may be −2 or −3 indicating that her bone mass is 20–30% below that of the average 30-year-old.

If one is having osteoporosis, chance of fracture (without added risk factors) is <5% in women below 50 years but >20% at the age of 65 years. Absolute risk increases further with additional risk factors, particularly with a previous fragility fracture. Overall fracture risk can be predicted by measurement or estimation of BMD at many skeletal sites.[23,24]

A Z-score compares bone density of woman to the average bone density of people of that age and gender. Z-score is a comparison of the BMD to an age-matched population score, the Z-score of −2 or lower is considered below the expected range for age. Score below the mean needs prompt careful scrutiny for coexisting problems (steroid therapy) that can contribute as a risk factor of osteoporosis. A Z-score is helpful in diagnosing secondary osteoporosis and is always used for children, young adults, women who are premenopausal, and men under age 50. If somebody has a very low Z-score (more than 2 standard deviations below other individuals of woman's age).

X-ray, CT scan, and MRI of the spine can be done if indicated.

Blood Chemistry

Full blood count, sedimentation rate, serum calcium, albumin, creatinine, phosphate, alkaline phosphatase, serum 25-hydroxyvitamin D, liver transaminases, thyroid function, and markers of bone turnover can be estimated if appropriate.

Those with abnormal initial findings may require additional testing to detect potentially reversible causes of osteoporosis. In addition, low BMD Z scores (age-matched comparison) identify individuals requiring further evaluation for secondary causes of osteoporosis.

Early diagnosis and quantification of bone loss and fracture risk are important because of the availability of therapies that can slow or even reverse the progression of osteoporosis.

■ SCREENING

The goal is to identify women who are at risk of sustaining a low trauma fracture and who benefit from intervention to minimize that risk of fracture. The US Preventive Services Task Force (USPSTF) found that, unlike men, in menopause women who do not have a history of previous fracture, drug therapy might reduce the risk of fracture. There are several screening methods that are discussed next.

Clinical Risk Factors

Assessment is an important method of screening to identify who are at risk. The WHO has defined osteoporosis based on dual-energy DEXA measurement. The relative risk of fracture increases as BMD decreases. But most fractures occur in women and men who do not have osteoporosis by DXA criteria. So clinical risk factors assessment has its own significance, clinical risk factors are independent of BMD. Validated risk factors are—advancing age, prior history of fracture, chronic steroid ingestion, low BMI, parenteral history of fracture, cigarette smoking, and excessive alcohol and sedentary habit. Most important risk factor for osteoporosis is history of fragility fracture.

But the criticism is only that clinical risk factors have shown poor sensitivity. About 50% women who begin menopause with an already low BMD have no clinical risk factors, so fracture risk assessment alone may not be too sensitive.

Though many studies showed low BMD is associated with increased risk of fracture,[25] methodologies for combining BMD with clinical risk factors to qualify fracture probability offer attractive alternative to relying on BMD testing alone.[26] Again, only clinical risk factors have shown poor sensitivity.

Nevertheless, univariate and multivariate analyses suggest that age, prior fracture history, and BMD are the strongest predictors of fracture risk. History of high or low trauma, nonspine fracture has elevated risk of subsequent fracture.[27]

FRAX

It is an assessment tool that allows estimation of 10 years' probability of hip fracture and major osteoporotic fracture with clinical factors.[28] The fracture risk (FRAX) of a patient over 10 years can be estimated as low (<10% in next 10 years), moderate (10–20% in next 10 years), or high (>20% in next 10 years) using known risk factors and femoral neck BMD. FRAX is based upon data from large observational data of men and women from different regions and ethnicity.[25] The FRAX is the most widely used model and has been validated in a large number of osteoporotic cohorts.[29] A country-specific FRAX is available for many countries (FRAX website: http://www.shef.ac.uk/FRAX/). But again, FRAX has very low sensitivity to predict the risk accurately. So, the clinician needs to individualize the risk on clinical judgment. FRAX does not appear to capture the changes in fracture risk associated with therapy and should not be used to monitor individuals who are on therapy.[30] In the menopause (MENOS) study, it was also shown that the FRAX model had limitation in some special cases such as women having diabetes mellitus, RA for fracture prediction with the first 10 years after menopause, performing no better than a single measurement of BMD.[31] It cannot determine the risk of other than hip site as FRAX algorithm includes femoral neck BMD (g/cm^2), BMD input from non-hip sites and other hip regions has not been validated with FRAX and is therefore, not recommended.[32]

A low BMD is a strong risk indicator for fracture risk, it is between the age of 50 and 60 years that gradient of risk for hip fracture is the highest as compared to that in older women.[15] The most commonly used bone measurement tests to screen osteoporosis are DXA of hip and lumbar spine. Therefore, greater reliance has to be placed on BMD in younger women, whereas in the elderly, risks will be better assessed by clinical factors, many of which increase with age. Several studies have shown that markers of bone turnover are able to predict rate of bone loss and osteoporotic fracture risk.[33]

The OFELY study showed the combination of a low BMD with a prior fracture and increased bone turnover markers (BTMs); (bone specific alkaline phosphatase) allows one to identify with increased fracture rate.[34] The FRAX tool should not be considered as a gold standard, but rather as a platform technology on which to build as new validated risk indicators become available. Notwithstanding, the present models provide an aid to enhance patient assessment by the integration of *clinical risk factors alone and/or in combination with BMD.*

Quantitative Ultrasonography

It does not measure the BMD but predicts risk. It is less expensive, less radiation exposure, and good in fracture prediction of femoral neck, hip, and spine.[35] Many studies showed that quantitative ultrasonography is as good as clinical risk factors predicting risk for osteoporosis.[36] But still now diagnosis and treatment depends on DXA.

Bone Turnover Markers

Bone turnover markers provide information of expected rates of bone loss and fracture risk that cannot be obtained from BMD.[37] These markers, measured in serum or urine, are not disease specific. They assess alteration in skeletal metabolism, regardless of the underlying causes. Combining BMD and BTM can improve fracture prediction. Significant changes in BTM can be seen during antiresorptive therapy after few weeks of treatment, whereas DEXA usually requires 1-2 years to identify significant changes. However, BTM could be used in clinical practice to assess the patient's adherence to treatment, and also provides the feedback on the effectiveness of the medication (Demas PD, IMPACT Study; ASBMR 2003).

Quantitative Computed Tomography

It measures volumetric BMD in mg/cm^2 which can provide information about bone mass, but these algorithms have yet to be validated on a large scale for osteoporosis screening.[38]

The most robust non-BMD risk factors are *age and previous fracture.*[39] Although clinical risk factors are predictive of bone density and fracture risk, they may not be as useful for predicting response to therapy for osteoporosis.[40]

Biochemical markers measurement can provide information about fracture risk but are not helpful against bone density measurement.[41]

Bone Mineral Density

It is used in conjunction with fracture risk assessment for osteoporosis screening.[42]

Who are the candidates for BMD screening?
According to the National Osteoporosis Foundation guidelines, 2014:
- Women ≥65 years, men >70 years, regardless of clinical risk factors

- Postmenopausal women and in menopausal transition with clinical risk factors[43]
- Condition associated with bone loss (e.g., RA)
- Adult with a fragility fracture
- Height loss of ≥2–4 cm.

■ TREATMENT OF OSTEOPOROSIS

Preventive

There is no current cure for osteoporosis. Prevention of fracture is the goal of treatment of osteoporosis. For everyone SD decrease in BMD at the hip, there is a 2.6-fold increase in the risk of hip fracture.[15] Thus, the prevention of low bone mass is directed to maximize peak bone mass and minimize the rate of loss with ultimate goal to make strong bone and prevent the fracture. Prevention of fall is another step to prevent fracture.

Osteoporosis treatment involves stopping further bone loss and strengthening bones that show signs of weakness.

Lifestyle Modification

- Nonpharmacological
- Pharmacological
- Fall prevention strategies
- Surgery, if indicated.

Recommended lifestyle:
- Ensuring adequate calcium and vitamin D intake
- Consuming a balance diet
- Performing weight-bearing and balance exercise regularly
- Avoiding tobacco use
- Limiting alcohol consumption
- Taking measures to avoid falls
- Considering use of hip protectors.

Lifestyle modification, i.e., regular exercise, nutritious diet, avoidance of sedentary habit and bone toxic agents, prevention of fall strategy are very important steps of prevention. Quitting smoking and moderation of alcohol ingestion are important strategies for risk reduction of osteoporosis.

Fall prevention strategies by improving:
- Poor lighting
- Unsafe stairways
- Irregular floor surfaces
- Home safety
- Removing throw rugs, low furniture
- Securing carpet edges
- Reducing clutter in the house

TABLE 2: Recommendation of calcium requirements in mg/day.		
Women over 50 years	1,200	2,000
Men (50–70 years)	1,000	2,000

- Bathroom-installing grab bars, using rubber mats
- Raising toilets seats
- Adequate lighting throughout the living spaces.

Dietary calcium needs to be encouraged as much as possible. Cheese, milk, yogurt, dark green vegetables, beans, orange, nuts, meat, fishes, almond, bread, and cereals are good source of calcium. Postmenopausal women should have dietary intake of calcium and vitamin D. Total intake of calcium is 1,200 mg/day (dietary supplement) is recommended for a postmenopausal woman.[44] The optimal intake of calcium and vitamin D is about 1,200 mg calcium (diet and supplement) and 800 IU of vitamin D daily for menopause women. It is advisable that atleast half of calcium requirement should come from the diet and the other half can be supplemented but total intake of calcium should not exceed beyond 2,000 mg/day to avoid cardiovascular side effects **(Table 2)**.

Most women need to take vitamin D supplementation, as it is difficult to achieve goals with diet alone. In celiac disease, gluten-free diet is advised to combat osteopenia. Protein intake should be ensured. Menopause ladies should also take protein. Recommendation of dietary protein is 1 g/kg/day.[45]

Practical Aspect of Calcium Use

$CaCO_3$ is cheap, better absorbed in acidic environment, and calcium should not be taken with antacid. Also, proton pump inhibitor or H2 blockers hinder calcium absorption. Each 1,250 mg $CaCO_3$ tablet contains 500 mg elemental calcium (40%). Calcium citrate should be a first-line supplementation in achlorhydria cases; 1,000 mg/day may be given in divided doses to avoid absorption plateau.

Side effects are risk of kidney stones and interference of absorption of iron and thyroid hormone.

Practical Points of Vitamin D Use

In meta-analysis, protective and effective daily dose of vitamin D is ≥800 IU (20 µg). Vitamin D helps in absorption of calcium from intestine.

Intermittent administration of large doses of vitamin D, e.g., ≥100,000 IU, is not advised (associated increased risk of fracture and falls). Vitamin D can be achieved from sunlight.

Exercise

Women with osteoporosis should exercise for at least 30 minutes three times per week. Most studies showed that exercise was associated with a reduced risk of hip fracture in older women; moderate weight-bearing exercise improves BMD at the spine and hip.[46] Observational cohort studies show that moderate weight-bearing exercise reduces the risk of hip fracture.[47] In a randomized controlled trial, 105 subjects by Kemmler W et al.[48] had study of women with exercise group and wolof women doing exercise without doing exercise group (exercise = 59 vs. control: n = 46) for 16-year follow-up, he showed the relative risk for overall low-trauma fractures 0.51 (95% CI: 0.23–0.97), p = 0.046) for the group of women doing exercise. Therefore, exercise should be the cornerstone of preventive strategies for osteoporosis and fracture.

Hormone Therapy

Women using menopausal hormone therapy (MHT) may prevent bone loss and fracture in the early postmenopausal period. In women having risk of osteoporosis, MHT can be continued with an acceptable risk-benefit ratio. The combined MHT estrogen–progestin therapy decreases the incidence of all fractures including vertebral and hip fractures even in women not at high risk. MHT most likely outweighs any risk and can be considered in women having risk factors for osteoporosis. In a meta-analysis of 57 trials (about 10,000 women), on an average, the increase in BMD after 2 years of estradiol/conjugated estrogens treated group was 6.8% in the spine and 4.1% in the hip and no difference was noted in results between prevention and treatment trial.[49] Since 2002, there have been more than 10 double blind trials lasting 2–3 years and were mainly using MHT therapy. The results from these trials showed that MHT increases bone mass density.[50]

Use of estrogen in older women showed an increase of 6% in spine BMD, 5% in total hip BMD, and 4% in femoral neck BMD compared to placebo.[51] Another study demonstrated increased spine BMD by 6.6%, femoral neck BMD 3.2%, and total hip BMD 3.1% compared to placebo. But to start, MHT in elderly women needs meticulous assessment of risks and benefits.

Third-generation New Hormone Preparations

Third-generation selective estrogen receptor modulators (SERMs), bazedoxifene, and lasofoxifene are approved in the European Union for the treatment of osteoporosis in menopausal women at increased risk of fracture. These have similar effect on bone as that of hormone estrogen. They help to maintain bone density and reduce risk of fracture, particularly in spine. It is unclear how long SERMs can be safely administered; many clinicians discontinue therapy at 8 years because of lack of safety data beyond that time frame.[52]

Since the decline in the use of estrogen therapy (ET) and concerns about the adverse effects of the progestin, there has been development of other

MHT-based preparations. The development of tissue selective estrogen complex that pairs conjugated estrogens with bazedoxifene that is a SERM. SERMs are an appropriate alternative for women who cannot take bisphosphonates due to side effects and those who cannot adhere to the dosing requirements for bisphosphonates.

Many trials have demonstrated the beneficial effect of raloxifene on BMD. In a meta-analysis of seven trials examining the effects of raloxifene versus placebo on BMD, raloxifene increased BMD of the lumbar spine of 1.8% and hip 2.1% after 2 years of treatment.[53] In another analysis,[54] 5 years postmenopause at baseline, 5 years of treatment with raloxifene 60 mg was associated with maintenance of BMD and reduced risk of developing fractures compared with placebo.

The North American Menopause Society recommends consideration of bone-specific medication in women with osteoporosis or low bone mass who have either a 10-year probability of a hip fracture of 3% or higher or a 10-year probability of a major osteoporosis-related fracture of 20% or higher [based on the US-adapted World Health Organization algorithm (FRAX)].

Ideal drugs for osteoporosis should have:
- Efficacy
- Scope of fracture protection
- Less adverse events
- Window of opportunity.

The National Osteoporosis Guideline Group 2017 approved treatments of osteoporosis for postmenopause women with calcium and vitamin D + drugs.

Antiresorptive drugs are bisphosphonates (alendronate, risedronate, ibandronate, and zoledronate), denosumab, calcitonin, MHT, and SERM. They work by slowing the resorption or breakdown the part of the remodeling cycle. Anabolic drugs act by stimulating the part of the remodeling process; more bone is formed than is taken away. These are parathyroid hormone, teriparatide, abaloparatide, and sclerostin inhibitors.

The drugs reduce the fragility fractures **(Table 3)**.

Alendronate, risedronate, zoledronic acid, and denosumab have the efficacy to reduce all sites fractures, and they are highly recommended. If patients are unable to take oral therapy, they may take teriparatide, denosumab or zoledronic acid as parenteral medicine. Side effects include nausea, abdominal pain, and heartburn-like symptoms. These are less likely to occur if the medicine is taken properly. IV bisphosphonate do not cause stomach upset but can cause fever, headache, and muscle pain.

Alendronate* can be used as—for prevention 5 mg/day, 35 mg/week and for treatment 10 mg/day, 70 mg/week; risedronate (for both preventive and therapeutic) 5 mg/day and 35 mg/week; ibandronate (for both preventive and therapeutic) 150 mg/month and treatment 3 mg IV every 3 months.

TABLE 3: Treatment of osteoporosis.

Intervention	Vertebral fracture	Non-vertebral fracture	Hip fracture
Alendronate	A	A	A
Ibandronate	A	A*	NAE
Risedronate	A	A	A
Zoledronic acid	A	A	A
Calcitriol	A	NAE	NAE
Denosumab	A	A	A
HRT	A	A	A
Raloxifene	A	NAE	NAE
Teriparatide	A	A	NAE

(A: grade A recommendation; NAE: not adequately evaluated; HRT: hormone replacement therapy)
* in subsets of patients only (post-hoc analysis).

Oral bisphosphonate should be taken at least 30 minutes before food with two full glasses of water and patient should remain upright, walking, standing, or sitting for at least 30 minutes. Patients need to be warned for few side effects such as hypocalcemia (18%), hypophosphatemia (10%), musculoskeletal pain, cramps, abdominal pain, dyspepsia, esophageal ulcer, gastritis, and visual disturbances. Food and Drug Administration (FDA) has warning of osteonecrosis of jaw (IV bisphosphonate).

Contraindications of bisphosphonates are hypocalcemia, hypersensitivity, and severe renal impairment (glomerular filtration rate ≤35 mL/min). There is some evidence that alendronate, risedronate, and teriparatide are effective in patients taking glucocorticoids.[55]

Denosumab

Denosumab is a human monoclonal antibody that acts on the key bone resorption mediator RANKL, thus inhibiting osteoclast formation and survival. It has been shown to increase BMD and reduce the incidence of fracture in postmenopausal women. It has similar or better bone density results and reduces the chance of all types of fractures. Denosumab 60 mg is delivered subcutaneously at 6 months interval. Because of the increased risk of fractures following discontinuation of therapy, continuing therapy or administration of another agent following discontinuation should be considered.[56,57]

Calcitonin is delivered in the nasal spray for daily use.

Anabolic Agents

Parathyroid hormone (teriparatide) and parathyroid-related protein analog (Abaloparatide) are available in injection form.

How to Monitor Treatment Result?

Baseline axial (spine and hip) DXA and then follow-up DXA every 1–2 years are done, follow-up ideally should be conducted in same facility with same machine.

How Long We should Continue Treatment?

FDA-approved teriparatide and abaloparatide treatment should be limited to no more than 2 years.

For oral bisphosphonates, consider a "bisphosphonate holiday", i.e., after 5 years of stability in moderate-risk patients, after 6–10 years of stability in high-risk patients and for IV zoledronic acid, consider a "drug holiday" after three annual doses in moderate-risk patients and after six annual doses in high-risk patients.

Follow-up

For women with T-score –2 to 2.49, without osteoporosis and not on therapy, BMD is done every 2 years. If T-score is –1.5 to 1.99, i.e., women with low bone mass, BMD is done at 3–5 years interval.

Women with normal or slight low bone mass (T-score: –1.01 to 1.49) should have repeat BMD at 15 years' interval. FRAX needs to be repeated at an interval of 5 years with further recommendation to perform a follow-up DXA earlier if the absolute fracture risk is close to the treatment threshold (3% for hip fracture and >20% for major osteoporotic fracture). Repeat BMD measurements may be most valuable for individual patients on therapy or to document stability of bone density in untreated patients with underlying clinical factors that might lead to accelerated bone loss.

Treatment failure may occur, so patients need to be strongly motivated for the use of drugs and they need to be counseled about the dangers for not taking the drugs. Usually it happens because of following factors:
- Poor compliance
- Calcium deficiency
- Vitamin D deficiency
- Comorbid conditions
- Using other medications
- Lack of efficacy of existing therapy.

Osteoporosis-related fractures of the hip, vertebra, and pelvis are a common cause of morbidity and mortality in postmenopause women.

FRAX helps in predicting patient's 10-year risk of hip or other major osteoporotic fracture and can help in guiding treatment decisions.

Fall prevention strategies can reduce the risk of fracture in patients with osteoporosis. All healthy adults should be counseled about measures to prevent osteoporosis, including adequate calcium and vitamin D intake, participating in weight-bearing exercise, avoiding tobacco and excess alcohol consumption, and having sun light.

Women should be screened for osteoporosis beginning at the age of 65 years. Screening for osteoporosis in men should be considered when risk factors are present. Appropriate screening intervals are controversial.

Women and men with osteoporosis should be offered pharmacologic therapy. Choice of therapy should be based on safety, cost, convenience, and other patient-related factors. Bisphosphonates are often first-line therapy based on efficacy, safety, and cost.

Hormone replacement therapy (HRT) with estrogen and progesterone helps increase calcium levels and prevent osteoporosis and fractures. ET restores postmenopausal bone remodeling to the same levels as at premenopause, leading to lower rates of bone loss.

■ KEY MESSAGES

- Osteoporosis is an emerging and long-lasting major public health issue, which is associated with significant morbidity and mortality and healthcare costs for menopause women.
- To prevent fall and subsequent and unfortunate fractures, it is essential for us to achieve a bone mass at an early age of 20–30 years.
- Effective drugs are available. MHT prevents bone loss or maintains bone health, but treatment and adherence to lifestyle modification and to MHT by patients are essentially suboptimal in real-world setting.
- BMD should be obtained routinely in all women of 65 years and younger women who have had a fragility fracture and premature menopause. Many of these patients will not lose bone mass if they have adequate intake of calcium and vitamin D, MHT, and regular exercise.
- Lifelong weight-bearing, strengthening, and balance training will help to achieve normal bone health. Timely osteoporosis identification, screening risk factors of osteoporosis, institution of proper lifestyle modification and effective drugs for treatment are cornerstone to prevent bone loss and fractures.
- If falls do occur in the elderly resulting fractures, surgery is to be allowed as early as possible.
- Postmenopausal women are at risk for osteoporosis and fractures.
- Weight-bearing and resistance exercise, limiting alcohol and caffeine intake, smoking cessation, and fall prevention strategies are part of a bone-healthy lifestyle used to manage postmenopausal osteoporosis.
- Supplements containing calcium and vitamin D are needed by many postmenopausal women because of an inadequate intake may accelerate bone loss.
- The osteoporosis drug therapy should take into consideration when osteoporosis is diagnosed.

- It depends on patient characteristics, patient's preference and drug efficacy, safety, route of administration, dosing frequency, convenience, cost, and potential for nonadherence.
- Bisphosphonates generally are preferred for the prevention and treatment of osteoporosis in postmenopausal women.
- Raloxifene, teriparatide, and calcitonin are alternatives.
- Denosumab, a fully human monoclonal immunoglobulin G(2) antibody is promising for prevention and treatment of postmenopausal osteoporosis.
- Health-system pharmacists can improve the management of osteoporosis in postmenopausal women by counseling them on a bone-healthy lifestyle and making recommendations for calcium and vitamin D supplements and osteoporosis medications to prevent or treat the disease.
- Bone mass density should be achieved in young adult life.

REFERENCES

1. Cauley JA. Public health impact of osteoporosis. J Gerontol A Biol Sci Med Sci. 2013;68(10):1243-51.
2. Cawthon PM. Gender differences in osteoporosis and fractures. Clin Orthop Relat Res. 2011;469(7):1900-5.
3. Johnell O. The socioeconomic burden of fractures: today and in the 21st century. Am J Med. 1997;103(2A):S20-6.
4. Baxter-Jones AD, Faulkner RA, Forwood MR, Mirwald RL, Bailey DA. Bone mineral accrual from 8 to 30 years of age: an estimation of peak bone mass. J Bone Miner Res. 2011;26(8):1729-39.
5. Tenenhouse A, Joseph L, Kreiger N, Poliquin S, Murray TM, Blondeau L, et al. CaMos Research Group. Canadian Multicentre Osteoporosis Study. Estimation of the prevalence of low bone density in Canadian women and men using a population-specific DXA reference standard: the Canadian Multicentre Osteoporosis Study (CaMos). Osteoporos Int. 2000;11(10):897-904.
6. Berger C, Goltzman D, Langsetmo L, Joseph L, Jackson S, Kreiger N, et al. Peak bone mass from longitudinal data: implications for the prevalence, pathophysiology, and diagnosis of osteoporosis. J Bone Miner Res. 2010;25(9):1948-57.
7. Miller GD, Weaver CM. Required versus optimal intakes: a look at calcium. J Nutr. 1994;124(8 Suppl):1404S-5S.
8. Matkovic V, Ilich JZ. Calcium requirements for growth: are current recommendations adequate? Nutr Rev. 1993;51(6):171-80.
9. Wyshak G, Frisch RE. Carbonated beverages, dietary calcium, the dietary calcium/phosphorus ratio, and bone fractures in girls and boys. J Adolesc Health. 1994;15(3):210-5.
10. Rannevik G, Jeppsson S, Johnell O, Bjerre B, Laurell-Borulf Y, Svanberg L. A longitudinal study of the perimenopausal transition: altered profiles of steroid and pituitary hormones, SHBG and bone mineral density. Maturitas. 1995;21(2):103-13.
11. Riggs BL, Melton III LJ. The prevention and treatment of osteoporosis. N Engl J Med. 1992;327(9):620-7.
12. Reeve J, Walton J, Russell LJ, Lunt M, Wolman R, Abraham R, et al. Determinants of the first decade of bone loss after menopause at spine, hip and radius. QJM. 1999;92(5):261-73.
13. Ravn P, Hetland ML, Overgaard K, Christiansen C. Premenopausal and postmenopausal changes in bone mineral density of the proximal femur measured by dual-energy X-ray absorptiometry. J Bone Miner Res. 1994;9(12):1975-80.

14. Falch JA, Sandvik L. Perimenopausal appendicular bone loss: a 10-year prospective study. Bone. 1990;11(6):425-8.
15. Marshall D, Johnell O, Wedel H. Meta-analysis of how well measures of bone mineral density predict occurrence of osteoporotic fractures. BMJ. 1996;312(7041):1254-9.
16. Svedbom A, Hernlund E, Ivergård M, Compston J, Cooper C, Stenmark J, et al. EU Review Panel of IOF. Osteoporosis in the European Union: a compendium of country-specific reports. Arch Osteoporos. 2013;8(1-2):137.
17. Hui SL, Slemenda CW, Johnston CC Jr. Baseline measurement of bone mass predicts fracture in white women. Ann Intern Med. 1989;111(5):355-61.
18. Shapses SA, Von Thun NL, Heymsfield SB, Ricci TA, Ospina M, Pierson RN Jr, et al. Bone turnover and density in obese premenopausal women during moderate weight loss and calcium supplementation. J Bone Miner Res. 2001;16(7):1329-36.
19. Finkelstein JS, Brockwell SE, Mehta V, Greendale GA, Sowers MR, Ettinger B, et al. Bone mineral density changes during the menopause transition in a multiethnic cohort of women. J Clin Endocrinol Metab. 2008;93(3):861-8.
20. Morin SN, Lix LM, Leslie WD. The importance of previous fracture site on osteoporosis diagnosis and incident fractures in women. J Bone Miner Res. 2014;29(7):1675-80.
21. Siris ES, Adler R, Bilezikian J, Bolognese M, Dawson-Hughes B, Favus MJ, et al. The clinical diagnosis of osteoporosis: a position statement from the National Bone Health Alliance Working Group. Osteoporos Int. 2014;25(5):1439-43.
22. Black DM, Cummings SR, Genant HK, et al. Axial and appendicular bone density predict fractures in older women. J Bone Miner Res. 1992;7:633.
23. Siris ES, Miller PD, Barrett-Connor E, Faulkner KG, Wehren LE, Abbott TA, et al. Identification and fracture outcomes of undiagnosed low bone mineral density in postmenopausal women: results from the National Osteoporosis Risk Assessment. JAMA. 2001;286(22):2815-22.
24. International Society for Clinical Densitometry. Adult positions. [online] Available from: https://iscd.org/learn/official-positions/adult-positions/ [Last accessed March, 2021].
25. Kanis JA, Borgstrom F, De Laet C, Johansson H, Johnell O, Jonsson B, et al. Assessment of fracture risk. Osteoporos Int. 2005;16(6):581-9.
26. Kanis JA, Oden A, Johnell O, Johansson H, De Laet C, Brown J, et al. The use of clinical risk factors enhances the performance of BMD in the prediction of hip and osteoporotic fractures in men and women. Osteoporos Int. 2007;18(8):1033-46.
27. Mackey DC, Lui LY, Cawthon PM, Bauer DC, Nevitt MC, Cauley JA, et al. Study of Osteoporotic Fractures (SOF) and Osteoporotic Fractures in Men Study (MrOS) Research Groups. High-trauma fractures and low bone mineral density in older women and men. JAMA. 2007;298(20):2381-8.
28. Leslie WD, Morin S, Lix LM, Johansson H, Oden A, McCloskey E, et al; Manitoba Bone Density Program. Fracture risk assessment without bone density measurement in routine clinical practice. Osteoporos Int. 2012;23(1):75-85.
29. WHO Fracture Risk Assessment Tool (FRAX). [online] Available from: http://www.shef.ac.uk/FRAX [Last accessed March, 2021].
30. Leslie WD, Lix LM. Can change in FRAX score be used to "treat to target"? A population-based cohort study. J Bone Miner Res. 2014;29(5):1074-80.
31. Kanis JA, Johansson H, Oden A, McCloskey EV. Guidance for the adjustment of FRAX according to the dose of glucocorticoids. Osteoporos Int. 2011;22(3):809-16.
32. Kanis JA, Johnell O, Oden A, Johansson H, McCloskey E. FRAX and the assessment of fracture probability in men and women from the UK. Osteoporos Int. 2008;19(4):385-97.
33. Vasikaran S, Eastell R, Bruyère O, Foldes AJ, Garnero P, Griesmacher A, et al. IOF-IFCC Bone Marker Standards Working Group. Markers of bone turnover for the

prediction of fracture risk and monitoring of osteoporosis treatment: a need for international reference standards. Osteoporos Int. 2011;22(2):391-420.
34. Sornay-Rendu E, Munoz F, Garnero P, Duboeuf F, Delmas PD. Identification of osteopenic women at high risk of fracture: the OFELY study. J Bone Miner Res. 2005;20(10):1813-9.
35. Marín F, González-Macías J, Díez-Pérez A, Palma S, Delgado-Rodríguez M. Relationship between bone quantitative ultrasound and fractures: a meta-analysis. J Bone Miner Res. 2006;21(7):1126-35.
36. Hodson J, Marsh J. Quantitative ultrasound and risk factor enquiry as predictors of postmenopausal osteoporosis: comparative study in primary care. BMJ. 2003;326(7401):1250-1.
37. Hansen MA, Overgaard K, Riis BJ, Christiansen C. Role of peak bone mass and bone loss in postmenopausal osteoporosis: 12 year study. BMJ. 1991;303(6808):961-4.
38. Baim S, Binkley N, Bilezikian JP, Kendler DL, Hans DB, Lewiecki EM, et al. Official Positions of the International Society for Clinical Densitometry and executive summary of the 2007 ISCD Position Development Conference. J Clin Densitom. 2008;11(1):75-91.
39. Yu EW. Screening of osteoporosis. [online] Available from: https://www.uptodate.com/contents/screening-for-osteoporosis-in-postmenopausal-women-and-men [Last accessed, March 2021].
40. Johnell O, Kanis JA, Black DM, Balogh A, Poor G, Sarkar S, et al. Associations between baseline risk factors and vertebral fracture risk in the Multiple Outcomes of Raloxifene Evaluation (MORE) Study. J Bone Miner Res. 2004;19(5):764-72.
41. Christiansen C, Riis BJ, Rødbro P. Prediction of rapid bone loss in postmenopausal women. Lancet. 1987;1(8542):1105-8.
42. Raisz LG. Clinical practice. Screening for osteoporosis. N Engl J Med. 2005;353(2):164-71.
43. US Preventive Services Task Force; Curry SJ, Krist AH, Owens DK, Barry MJ, Caughey AB, Davidson KW, et al. Screening for osteoporosis to prevent fractures: US Preventive Services Task Force Recommendation Statement. JAMA. 2018;319(24):2521-31.
44. Institute of Medicine. (2011). Report at a Glance, Report Brief: Dietary reference intakes for calcium and vitamin D. [online] Available from: https://www.nap.edu/resource/13050/Vitamin-D-and-Calcium-2010-Report-Brief.pdf [Last accessed, March 2021].
45. Holick MF. Vitamin D deficiency. N Engl J Med. 2007;357(3):266-81.
46. Shanb AA, Youssef EF. The impact of adding weight-bearing exercise versus nonweight bearing programs to the medical treatment of elderly patients with osteoporosis. J Family Community Med. 2014;21(3):176-81.
47. Feskanich D. Exercise to prevent fracture. JAMA. 2002;288(18):2300-6.
48. Kemmler W, Bebenek M, Kohl M, von Stengel S. Exercise and fractures in postmenopausal women. Final results of the controlled Erlangen Fitness and Osteoporosis Prevention Study (EFOPS). Osteoporos Int. 2015;26(10):2491-9.
49. Wells G, Tugwell P, Shea B, Guyatt G, Peterson J, Zytaruk N, et al. Meta-analyses of therapies for postmenopausal osteoporosis. V. Meta-analysis of the efficacy of hormone replacement therapy in treating and preventing osteoporosis in postmenopausal women. Endocr Rev. 2002;23(4):529-39.
50. Gallagher JC. Effect of estrogen on bone. In: Favus MJ (Ed). Primer on the Metabolic Bone Diseases and Disorders of Mineral Metabolism, 5th edition. Washington, DC: American Society for Bone and Mineral Research; 2006. pp. 327-30.
51. Gallagher JC, Fowler SE, Detter JR, Sherman SS. Combination treatment with estrogen and calcitriol in the prevention of age-related bone loss. J Clin Endocrinol Metab. 2001;86(8):3618-28.

52. Black DM, Rosen CJ. Clinical Practice. Postmenopausal Osteoporosis. N Engl J Med. 2016;374(3):254-62.
53. Cranney A, Tugwell P, Zytaruk N, Robinson V, Weaver B, Adachi J, et al. Osteoporosis Methodology Group and The Osteoporosis Research Advisory Group. Meta-analyses of therapies for postmenopausal osteoporosis. IV. Meta-analysis of raloxifene for the prevention and treatment of postmenopausal osteoporosis. Endocr Rev. 2002;23(4):524-8.
54. Jolly EE, Bjarnason NH, Neven P, Plouffe L Jr, Johnston CC Jr, Watts SD, et al. Prevention of osteoporosis and uterine effects in postmenopausal women taking raloxifene for 5 years. Menopause. 2003;10(4):337-44.
55. Adami G, Saag KG. Glucocorticoid-induced osteoporosis: 2019 concise clinical review. Osteoporos Int. 2019;30(6):1145-56.
56. Qaseem A, Forciea MA, McLean RM. Denberg TD. Treatment of low bone density or osteoporosis to prevent fractures in men and women: a clinical practice guideline update from the American College of Physicians. Ann Intern Med. 2017;166(11):818-39.
57. Tsourdi E, Langdahl B, Cohen-Solal M, Aubry-Rozier B, Eriksen EF, Guañabens N, et al. Discontinuation of Denosumab therapy for osteoporosis: A systematic review and position statement by ECTS. Bone. 2017;105:11-7.

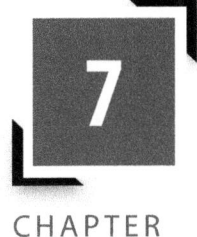

Cardiovascular Health and Menopause

CHAPTER

■ INTRODUCTION

Menopause means the permanent cessation of menstruation at the end of the reproductive life (average age 51). It may produce some bothersome symptoms such as hot flushes, night sweats, palpitation, body ache, joint pain, and genitourinary syndrome of menopause (GSM) but it can also be the start of new and rewarding phase of women's life and the golden opportunity to guard against major health risks such as cardiovascular disease (CVD) and osteoporosis. CVD risk rises for everyone as women grow older, but beyond menopause, risk of CVD increases dramatically and more than their counter partner. In young women, who have early menopause and not taking menopausal hormone therapy (MHT), their risk of CVD is also very high. Coronary heart disease (CHD) is the single most common cause of death of women and significant cause of disability. CVD has become the leading killer of women across the world.[1] In fact, one-third of all deaths in women after the age of 50 occur due to CVD that include CHD, myocardial infarction, and valvular diseases. The study of Rupal Dosi et al. showed CVD are more common in postmenopausal women of 50–55 years as compared to those not yet achieved menopause.[2] They emphasized menopause as an independent risk factor for heart disease. As estrogen is believed to have a positive effect on inner layer of vessels, decline of estrogen is associated with thickening of endometrium which becomes the risk factor for CVD. There are also other risk factors of CVD, those are smoking, diabetes, raised BP, high low-density lipoprotein (LDL), obesity, sedentary lifestyle, and family history of the CVD. Women are not very aware of these risk factors rather they are very concerned about breast cancer but the incidence of CVD is nine times more than breast cancer[3] and so CVD is now becoming the global health issue. Therefore, women need to adopt the strategies to prevent CVD and maintain a good healthy heart so menopause is the window opportunity for prevention of CVD and encourage a proactive approach for future well-being.[4] Estrogen and testosterone are involved in CVD and these are related to endothelial function, vascular tone and cardiac function.[5] **Figure 1** shows diminution of estrogen level in blood declines after menopause.[6]

We know that estrogen keeps the blood vessels flexible. It increases good cholesterol and decreases the peripheral resistance. Estrogen prevents atherosclerosis **(Fig. 2)** and inflammatory changes and is more lipids friendly [high-density lipoprotein (HDL) > LDL], thus preventing cardiovascular

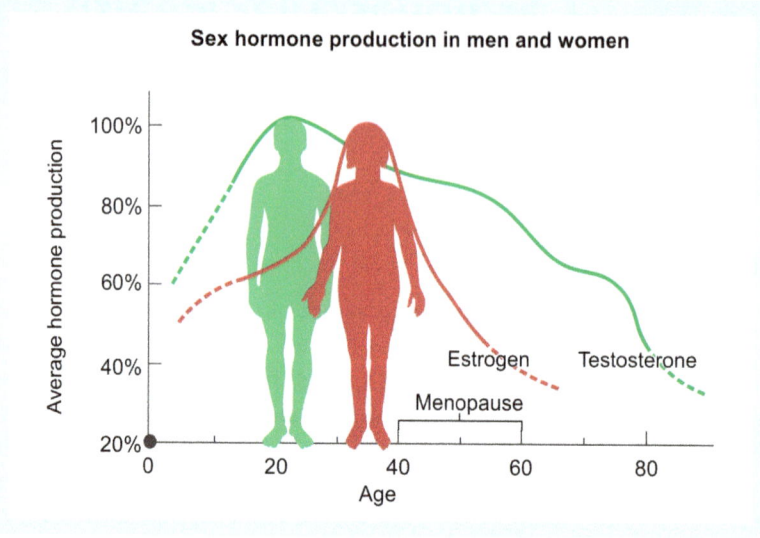

Fig. 1: Reduced hormone after menopause.[6]

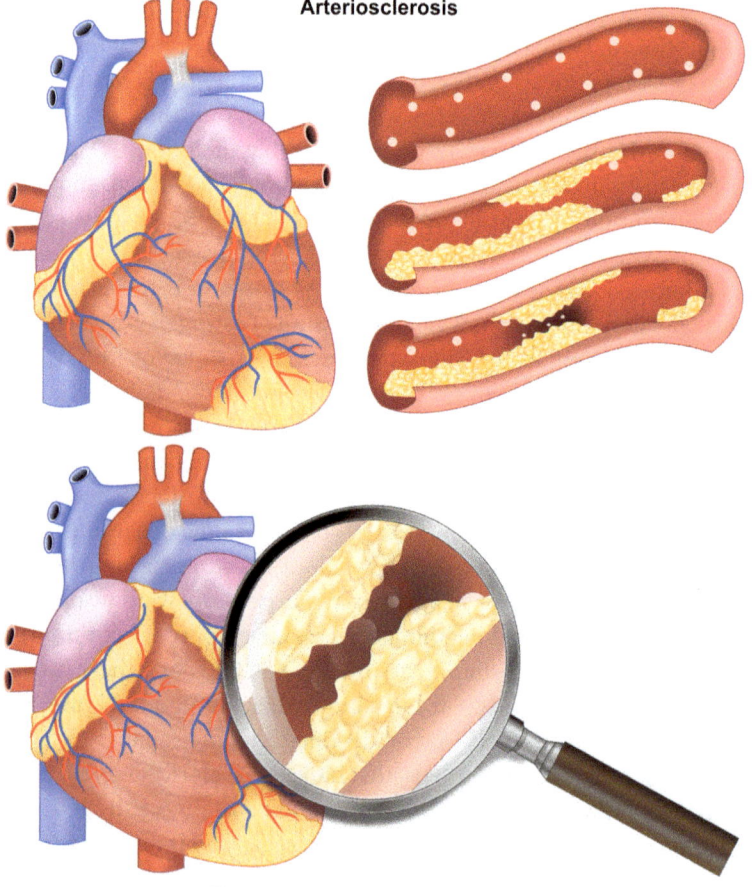

Fig. 2: Normal heart and atheroma.

events. Estrogen enhances nitric oxide (NO) and prostacyclin release, which are potent vasodilators. In addition it reduces the production of endothelial, derived platelets factors, and angiotensin that are vasoconstrictors. Most importantly estrogen reduces tumor necrosis factor (TNF) alpha and increases prostacyclin I which reduces oxidative stress and platelet activation.

■ IMPACT OF MENOPAUSE

Decline in the levels of endogenous estrogen at menopause, increases the risk of vasomotor symptoms, osteoporosis, CVDs, and dementia **(Fig. 3)**.

Menopause negatively impacts the metabolic system too such as changes body fat distribution **(Figs. 4A and B)** from gynoid to an android pattern (pear to apple shape). Visceral fat is deposited in the upper abdomen, which is detrimental for CVD.

Menopause increases blood pressure, sympathetic tone, endothelial dysfunction, vascular inflammation, and cardiovascular events correlate with loss of endothelial dysfunction.[7] Menopause negatively impacts the metabolic system such as changes body fat distribution from gynoid to an android pattern,[8] reduced glucose tolerance, increased insulin resistance[9] and it leads to cardiovascular complications. Menopause is associated with

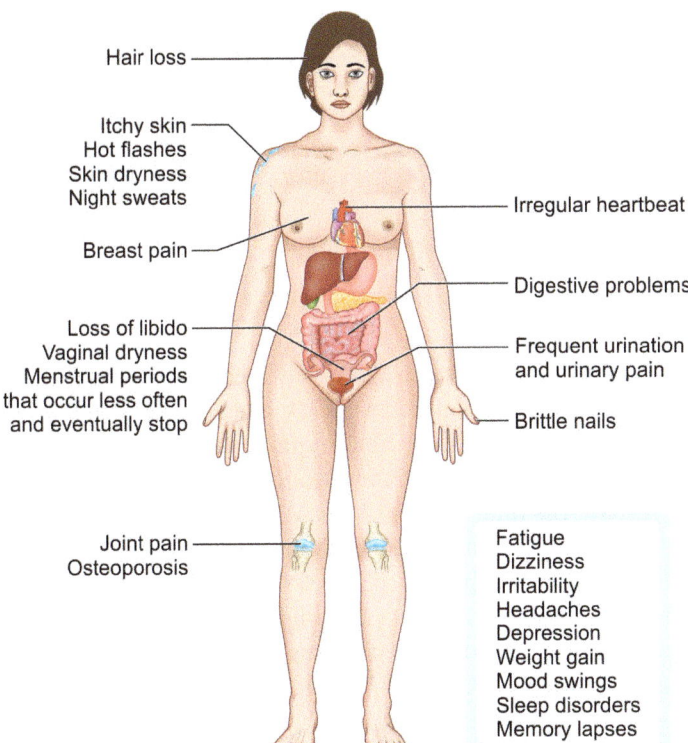

Fig. 3: Effects of menopause.

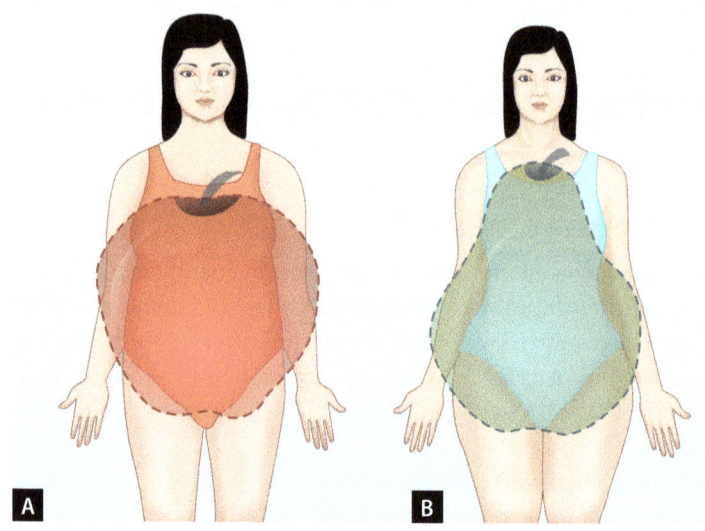

Figs. 4A and B: Changes of fat distribution.

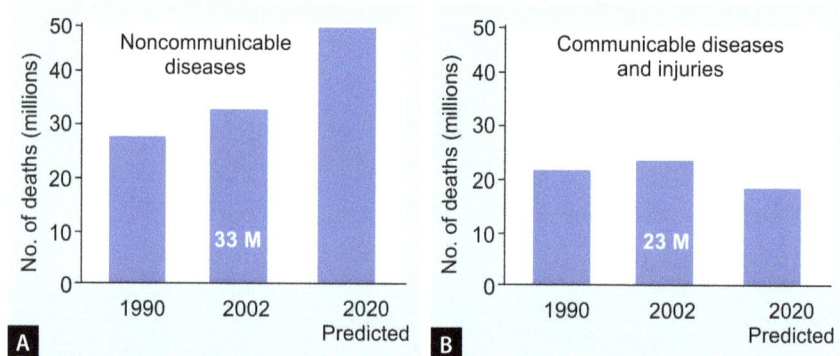

Figs. 5A and B: Death patterns of noncommunicable and communicable diseases.[10]

decrease in HDL and increase LDL that may mediate higher CHD.[10] Women suffering from vasomotor symptoms are at greater risk of CVD.

Women of any age with vasomotor symptoms have a worse cardiovascular risk profile (increased risk of CVD, CHD, or ischemic stroke) compared with women without vasomotor symptoms. Women experiencing vasomotor symptoms have significantly higher systolic and diastolic blood pressures, higher circulating total cholesterol levels and a higher body mass index than their counterparts with no symptoms. It is reported that women will die more from noncommunicable diseases in upcoming years and CVD will be the main killer **(Figs. 5A and B)**.[11] Therefore, all women need to be aware about the noncommunicable diseases including the risks of CVD at their late age.

ROLE OF MENOPAUSAL HORMONE TREATMENT

The Women's Health Initiative (WHI) conducted two placebo-controlled trials in women aged 50-79 and showed increased risk of CHDs and stroke in women with hormone. Generally, estrogens lower LDL, raise HDL, and increase triglycerides.

Menopausal hormone treatment can be useful in controlling the vasomotor symptoms beside that it exerts a bone sparing effect, preventing lower bone mass density and reduces fracture risk for menopausal women.[12] However, the WHI study demonstrated a significant increase in CVD and stroke with after 5.2 years of estrogen + progestin use.[13] But there was a huge limitation of the WHI study of 2002, to this day, the results are still being debated, reinterpreted, reanalyzed and in many cases it was misinterpreted. WHI trials primarily designed to test whether MHT prevented the occurrence of CHD, stroke and breast cancer in postmenopausal women who were ≥ 10 years postmenopause women and mostly asymptomatic. Mean age of enrollment (n = 16,608) was 63 years, with only 33% of the study population aged 50-59 years and 22% aged 70 years or older. Evaluation was done with only one dose of hormone and one route of administration. So WHI study was not well-designed and not powered to investigate consequences of MHT in women less than 60 years. Findings were biased and reported for the total study group than generalized all postmenopausal women. Therefore, in 2013, the whole study was reanalyzed which clearly showed association between MHT and CVD risk is influenced in women by the factors age and time since menopause. In fat women, it is seen from recent Cochrane analysis, women within 10 years of menopause using MHT had reduction of cardiovascular mortality of 0.52 (95% CI 0.29-0.96).[14] But in observational studies of women with and without existing CHD, the use of postmenopausal hormone therapy is associated with a reduced risk of CHD events.[15] Women who initiated hormone therapy closer to menopause tended to have reduced CHD risk compared with the increase in CHD risk among women more distant from menopause.[16] The Danish Osteoporosis study (DOPS) by their 16 years follow-up showed, there were significant reduction in mortality and hospitalization for myocardial infarction and congestive heart failure.[17] Benefits of MHT depend on timing of initiation, dose and duration of the MHT.[18] Estrogen in MHT is protective against atherogenesis in women who have not developed atheroma (*see* **Fig. 2**) but starting hormones in women who already have atheroma is not useful.[19] MHT with estrogen in older women did not show cardiovascular benefits.[20] Within 10 years of menopause MHT has higher benefits-risk ratio for cardiovascular health and menopause women.[21] Meta-analysis of randomized controlled trials (RCTs) showed significant reduction of CHD and mortality, if MHTs are taken under the age of 60.[22] Finish study showed using MHT causes 19 fewer deaths and 7 fewer stroke deaths per 1,000 women.[23] Timing hypothesis is important.

Danish study showed that early starting of MHT is associated with significant reduction of risk of CVD. ELITE trial showed estrogen arm had significant slower progression of coronary media thickness among women who initiated MHT less than 6 years after menopause.[24] The National Institute for Health and Care Excellence (NICE) states, women should know that CVD risk factors such as hypertension, diabetes, are not contraindication for MHT provided they are well-controlled. Avoiding MHT may be detrimental to CVD. Studies showed that increased mortality was found in the first year of stoppage of MHT.[25] The Indian Menopause Society (IMS) updated recommendation on postmenopausal hormone therapy stated that MHT markedly reduces the risk of diabetes, through improved insulin resistance, and it has positive effects on other relative risks factors for CVD such as the lipid profile and metabolic syndrome.[26] In women less than 60 years old, recently menopausal, without prevalent CVD the initiation of MHT does not cause harm and may reduce cardiovascular morbidities and mortalities. Continuation of MHT beyond the age of 60 should be decided as a part of overall risk-benefit analysis.

Low dose MHT is unlikely harmful. Regarding progestin better to avoid if necessary, microionized progesterone seems to have a neutral or beneficial effects on blood pressure in postmenopausal women.[27] Beneficial effects of estrogen are not attenuated when they are with natural progesterone, some synthetic progestins such as medroxyprogesterone acetate (MPA), which blunts the increase of HDL by estrogen. Progesterone also has beneficial effects in preventing the growth and movement of cells involved in the formation of arteriosclerotic plaques and relaxing arterial smooth muscle via enhancement of NO from the endothelium. Natural progesterone has a neutral effect on lipid and glucose metabolism and on vascular tone. MPA at high doses for cyclical administration abolishes the beneficial effect of estrogen. But when MPA is used at lower doses incontinuous combined regimen, no effect is observed. Androgen-derivative progestins (norethisterone acetate) have a detrimental effect. Dydrogesterone (devoid of androgenic effect) does not reverse the beneficial effect of estrogen.[28] Drospirenone has been shown significantly lowers BP in hypertension and provides positive effects on cardiovascular profile.[29] MHT reduces chronic disabilities but US Preventive Services Task Force (USPSTF) did not find any significant role of estrogen to prevent chronic diseases. So MHT is not to be given just for prevention of chronic conditions in postmenopausal women.[30]

Statin does not help in primary prevention of CVD in women,[31] total beneficial effect of aspirin as primary prevention in women is no longer deemed positive.[32] Maintaining good heart health is of utmost importance; so regular heart health screening is the cornerstone to prevent CVD. As estrogen deficiency during menopause increases the risk hypertension, diabetes, dyslipidemia,[33] regular exercise, eating healthy diet and staying positive are most important strategies to prevent heart diseases. Along with that optimum control of comorbidities are required. But women need to start MHT earlier in order to get the maximum cardiovascular protection. Women with premature ovarian insufficiency (POI) is the condition when ovaries stop to work before the age of 40 years, early menopause and women within 10 years of menopause can potentially gain significant improvements in their cardiovascular and general health. Early menopause means when menopause occurs before the age of 45 years. The side effects of MHT are very small in absolute number, especially in younger women, where the overall benefits of MHT is high, also MHT manifests in reduce mortality.[34] The Global Consensus statements of 2013, issued by all menopausal societies is consistent with Cochrane Review including evidences from randomized trial and meta-analysis state that standard dose of estrogen alone may decrease CHD and all-cause mortality in women younger than 60 years of age and within 10 years of menopause.[35]

■ PREVENTION OF CARDIOVASCULAR DISEASES

Cardiovascular Disease Screen

The World Health Organization (WHO) developed risk prediction chart from best available mortality and risk data of those from low and middle income countries population (LMIC). They are meant to be used in LMIC, where refined risk prediction charts do not exist. At present these charts are necessarily crude but are safe and useful tools for guiding the prevention and management decision or individual.

When are the Charts Useful for Stratifying Risks

Charts are useful for stratifying risk for people with BP <160/100 mm Hg or blood cholesterol <8 mmol/L or uncomplicated diabetes.

For example, by using the charts, person X and Y who have similar BP and blood cholesterol levels can be correctly assessed for their risk of development of heart attack or stroke, as described in **Table 1**.

Person X needs lifestyle modification and must adopt preventive strategies, and may need drugs only if risks are not eliminated during follow-up consultation.

Person Y needs intensive lifestyle interventions and may need drug treatment if risk persists.

Cardiovascular disease is the major killer in women, more than men, unfortunately only 9% of menopause women knew about menopause

	Risk factors profiles	10 years risk of heart attack or stroke
Male X, 50 years	SBP 140 mm Hg TC 7 mm/L, non-smokers, no diabetes	10–20%
Male Y, 50 years	SBP 140 mm Hg, TC 7 mmol/L, smoker and diabetic	>4%

TABLE 1: Risk prediction using charts.

(SBP: systolic blood pressure; TC: triglycerides)

and only 3% women are aware of relation of menopause and CVD. Many women have no knowledge of risk factors for CVD due to lack of awareness.[36] A healthy lifestyle goes a long way in preventing CVD in women.

Healthy lifestyle, optimum diet and exercise are the corner stone to prevent the CVD. In addition, MHT can play a significant role. MHT increases HDL cholesterol and decreases LDL compared to statins, which actually have little effect on these levels.

Diet has a vital role. Women need to avoid salty, oily food. They should cut down fatty food and maintain optimum body weight. American Heart Association recommends eating a dietary pattern that emphasizes—fruits, vegetables, whole grains **(Fig. 6)**, low fat dairy products, poultry, fish, and nuts, while limiting red meat and sugary foods and beverages.

Healthy lifestyle not only means diet control but it includes avoiding or quitting smoking, maintaining healthy body weight and doing regular exercise. Healthy diet, treatment and control of medical conditions such as hypertension, diabetes, and hyperlipidemia are very important steps to prevent CVD. Exploring what brings pleasure, having positive thoughts, loving her and reviving not retiring from sex life are other additional elements to improve mental health and thereby prevent CVD.

Exercise

Exercise (it's never too late to start; menopause is perfect time to do more activity into our life rather looking back mournfully). Exercise includes aerobic, muscle strengthening, flexibility, breathing and balance. Women should exercise at last 150 min/week up to 300 min/week depending on the individual's need. To prevent CVDs women should do 30 min/day of moderate intense physical activity mostly 5 days/week.

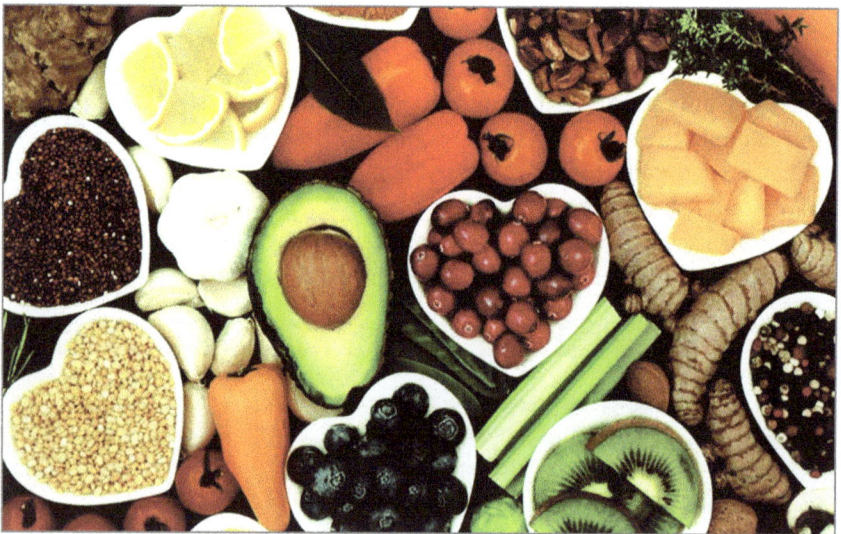

Fig. 6: American Heart Association healthy diet for women to reduce CVD risks.

Muscle strengthening activities should be done 2 days/week. They should do exercise 60 min/day to prevent weight gain. Walking, cycling, swimming and dancing are good common exercises.

Kegel exercise should be done to maintain the pelvic floor strength. Healthy women can probably undertake such a program without medical screening. Those who have any medical problems or symptoms (e.g., chest pain, dyspnea, syncope) should be evaluated thoroughly before beginning such a program.

Menopausal Hormone Therapy

Actually menopause is not a disease it is a natural event of life, so Dr Goldberg said, "It's important for women, as they approach menopause, to really take stock of their health."[36] During this time women may get some leisure, may concentrate to look after herself. Already the beneficial effects of estrogen therapy is been stated earlier. If MHT is administered in postmenopausal women for any symptoms they exert their utmost benefits for the cardiovascular health. But MHT needs to be administered below the age of 60 years or within 10 years of menopause.

■ KEY MESSAGES

- Prevention of CVD in menopause women should be started early in midlife with optimum diet and physical activities.
- Menopause is the time to have checkups including assessment of cardiovascular risks and to start a healthy lifestyle.
- Menopausal hormone therapy is not recommended for primary cardiovascular disease prevention. But women need to start MHT earlier in order to get the maximum cardiovascular protection.
- Women with POI, early menopause and women within 10 years of menopause can potentially gain significant improvements with MHT in their cardiovascular and general health. MHT is beneficial for cardiovascular health.
- Women using MHT for any reason during window period, maximum benefits of cardiovascular profile are obtained. For women with POI, MHT needs to be used earlier and should be continued till the age of natural menopause.
- Deficiency of estrogen and gradual aging affect vessel wall at different stages of menopause transition. Menopause is the time to have a checkup including assessment of CVD risk with prompt intervention if necessary.
- There are no related dangers associated with taking MHT and there are indications of some possible benefits on menopause women. Consideration of MHT should be part of an overall strategy including lifestyle recommendations regarding diet, exercise, smoking cessation and safe levels of alcohol consumption for maintaining the health of peri- and postmenopausal women.

- Menopausal hormone therapy must be individualized and tailored according to symptoms, the need for prevention, personal and family history, results of investigations and each woman's preferences and expectations need to be considered.

REFERENCES

1. Mosca L. The role of hormone replacement therapy in the prevention of postmenopausal heart disease. Arch Intern Med. 2000;160(15):2263-72.
2. Dosi R, Bhatt N, Shan P. Cirrhosis: an unusual presentation of sickle cell disease. J Clin Diagn Res. 2014;8(2):62.
3. Heather C, Christine W. Menopause, cholesterol and cardiovascular disease. Eur Cardiol Rev. 2008;4(1):17-20.
4. Stuenkel CA, Davis SR, Gompel A, Lumsden MA, Murad MH, Pinkerton JV, et al. Treatment of symptoms of the menopause: an endocrine society clinical practice guideline. J Clin Endocrinol Metab. 2015;100(11):3975-4011.
5. Mendelsohn ME, Karas RH. Molecular and cellular basis of cardiovascular gender differences. Science. 2005;308(5728):1583-7.
6. Yang Y. The importance of testosterone in women's health: unleash the power of nature. Emp Herbs. 2018.
7. Hamburg NM, Keyes MJ, Larson MG, Ramachandan S, Schnabel VR, Pryder MM, et al. Cross-sectional relations of digital vascular function to cardiovascular risk factors in the Framingham Heart Study. Circulation. 2008;117(19);2467-74.
8. Keller C, Larkey L, Distefano JK, Robillard EA, Veres S, Al-Zadjali M, et al. Perimenopausal obesity. J Womens Health. 2010;19(5):987-96.
9. Writing Group on behalf of Workshop Consensus Group. Aging, menopause, cardiovascular disease and HRT. International Menopause Society Consensus Statement. Climacteric. 2009;12(5):368-77.
10. Mozaffarian D, Rimm EB, Herrington DM. Dietary fats, carbohydrate, and progression of coronary atherosclerosis in postmenopausal women. Am J Clin Nutr. 2004;80(5):1175-84.
11. Yach D, Hawkes C, Gould CL, Hofman KJ. The global burden of chronic diseases: overcoming impediments to prevention and control. JAMA. 2004;291(21):2616-22.
12. Torgerson DJ, Bell-Syer SE. Hormone replacement therapy and prevention of nonvertebral fractures: a meta-analysis of randomized trials. JAMA. 2001;285(22):2891-7.
13. JoAnn Manson MD, Chelebowski RT, Stefanic ML, Aragak AK, Rossouw JE, Ross L. Menopausal hormone therapy and health outcomes during intervention and extended postsopping phase of the Women's Health Initiative randomized trials. JAMA. 2013;310(13):1353-68.
14. Boardman HM, Hartley L, Eisinga A, Main C, Roque I, Figuls M, et al. Hormone replacement on cardiovascular therapy disease post-menopausal women. Cochrane Database Syst Rev. 2015;3:CD002229.
15. Barrett-Connor E, Grady D. Hormone replacement therapy, heart disease, and other considerations. Annu Rev Public Health. 1998;19:55-72.
16. Rossouw JE, Prentice RL, Manson JE, Wu L, Barad D, Barnabei VM, et al. Postmenopausal hormone therapy and risk of cardiovascular disease by age and years since menopause. JAMA. 2007;297(13):1465-77.
17. Schierbeck LL, Rejnmark L, Tofteng CL, Stilgren L, Eiken P, Mosekilde L, et al. Effect of hormone replacement therapy on cardiovascular events in recently post-menopausal women: randomised trial. BMJ. 2012;345:e6409.
18. L'Hermite M. HRT optimization, using transdermal estradiol plus micronized progesterone, a safer HRT. Climacteric. 2013;16(Suppl 1):44-53.

19. Santen RJ. Use of cardiovascular age for assessing risks and benefits of menopausal hormone therapy. Menopause. 2017;24(5):589-95.
20. Rossouw JE, Anderson GL, Prentice RL, LaCroix AZ, Kooperberg C, Stefanick ML, et al. Risks and benefits of estrogen plus progestin in healthy postmenopausal women: principal results from the Women's Health Initiative randomized controlled trial. JAMA. 2002;288(3):321-33.
21. NICE. (2015). Menopause: diagnosis and management. [online] Available from: https://www.nice.org.uk/guidance/ng23/resources/menopause-diagnosis-and-management-pdf-1837330217413 [Last accessed February, 2021].
22. Salpeter SR, Cheng J, Thabane L, Buckley NS, Salpeter EE. Bayesian meta-analysis of hormone therapy and mortality in younger women. Ann Intern Med. 2009; 122:1016-22.
23. Mikkola TS, Tuomikoski P, Lyytinen H, Korhonen P, Hoti F, Vattulainen P, et al. Estradiol-based postmenopausal hormone therapy and risk of cardiovascular and all-cause mortality. Menopause. 2015;22(9):976-83.
24. Hodis HN, Mack WJ, Henderson VW, Shoupe D, Budoff MJ, Hwang-Levine J, et al. Vascular effects of early versus late postmenopausal treatment with estradiol. N Engl J Med. 2016;374(13):1221-31.
25. Mikkola TS, Tuomikoski P, Lyytinen H, Korhonen P, Hoti F, Vattulainen P, et al. Increased cardiovascular mortality risk in women discontinuing postmenopausal hormone therapy. J Clin Endocrinol Metab. 2015;100(12):4588-94.
26. Board of the International Menopause Society, Pines A, Sturdee DW, Birkhäuser MH, Schneider HP, Gambacciani M, et al. IMS updated recommendations on postmenopausal hormone therapy. Climacteric. 2007;10(3):181-94.
27. Honisett SY, Pang B, Stojanovska L, Sudhir K, Komesaroff PA. Progesterone does not influence vascular function in postmenopausal women. J Hypertens. 2003; 21(6):1145-9.
28. Gambacciani M, Monteleone P, Vitale C, Silvestri A, Fini M, Genazzani AR, et al. Dydrogesterone does not reverse the effects of estradiol on endothelium-dependant vasodilation in postmenopausal women: a randomised clinical trial. Maturitas. 2002;43(2):117-23.
29. Rosano GM, Vitale C, Marazzi G, Volterrani M. Menopause and cardiovascular disease: the evidence. Climacteric. 2007;10(Suppl 1):19-24.
30. US Preventive Services Task Force, Grossman DC, Curry SJ, Owens DK, Barry MJ, Davidson KW, et al. Hormone Therapy for the Primary Prevention of Chronic Conditions in Postmenopausal Women: US Preventive Services Task Force Recommendation Statement. JAMA. 2017;318(22):2224-33.
31. Nilsson S, Mölstad S, Karlberg C, Karlsson JE, Persson LG. No connection between the level of exposition to statins in the population and the incidence/mortality of acute myocardial infarction: an ecological study based on Sweden's municipalities. J Negat Results Biomed. 2011;10(1):6.
32. Halvorsen S, Andreotti F, Ten Berg JM, Cattaneo M, Coccheri S, Marchioli R, et al. Aspirin therapy in primary cardiovascular disease prevention: a position paper of the European Society of Cardiology working group on thrombosis. J Am Coll Cardiol. 2014;64(3):319-27.
33. Atsma F, Bartelink ML, Grobbee DE, vander Schouw YT. Postmenopausal status and early menopause as independent risk factors for cardiovascular disease: a meta-analysis. Menopause. 2006;13(2):265-79.
34. Salpeter SR, Walsh JM, Greyber E, Ormiston TM, Salpeter EE. Mortality associated with hormone replacement therapy in younger and older women: a meta-analysis. LJ Gen Intern Med. 2004;19(7):791-804.
35. de Villiers TJ, Gass ML, Haines CJ, Hall JE, Lobo RA, Pierroz DD, et al. Global consensus statement on menopausal hormone therapy. Climacteric. 2013;16(2):203-4.
36. Tandon VR, Mahajan A, Sharma S, Sharma A. Prevalence of cardiovascular risk factors in postmenopausal women: A rural study. J Mid Life Health. 2010;1(1):26-9.

CHAPTER 8

Brain, Cognition and Menopause

■ INTRODUCTION

Menopause is the permanent cessation of menstruation and the end of women's reproductive capacity.[1] Several health issues are associated with the progression of menopause. Memory problems and menopause go side-by-side but other health issues such as low bone mineral density, mood disorders, vaginal dryness, muscle-joint pain are also important. Many patient experience "brain fog" or cognitive decline, i.e., problem with memory, concentration, confusion, problem with thinking and learning along with disturbed sleep, anxiety, depression, sexual dysfunction, vasomotor irregularities.[2] Whether menopause triggers this "brain fog" or impaired cognition is still a matter of controversy. The changes occurring during and after menopause are due to changes in various hormones such as follicular stimulating hormone (FSH)[3] and decreased estrogen. The exact effect of estrogen and progesterone loss on the brain is not well-understood. It is believed that estrogen may help the neurotransmitter systems that send signals in brain areas involved in memory and information processing. Many researchers also think that estrogen promotes the growth and survival of neurons, the cells that send electrical impulses. These impulses serve as messages that are crucial for making brain and nervous system work properly.

Estrogen influences hippocampus and prefrontal cortex, which promotes cognitive functions (verbal memory and executive function).[4] Estrogen directly affects the brain function by having an effect on the vascular and the immune system.[5] Potential association of menopausal hormonal changes with brain function may therefore be approached in two ways: (1) directly—effects on neural cells and systems, and (2) indirectly—effects of hormonal changes on evidenced functions, mainly cognition and mood.[6]

Fluctuation in estrogen and progesterone level and decline in estrogen level are potentially relevant to cognitive changes occurring during premature menopause.

In addition the menopausal cardinal symptoms, hot flashes, night sweats, sleep disturbance, depression, anxiety, and mood swing can leave one feeling more fatigue and indirectly more cognitive impairment.

There is increasing evidence that menopausal changes can have an impact on women's cognition and potentially, and the future development of dementia. In particular, the role of reduced levels of estrogen in postmenopausal changes has been linked to an increased risk of developing dementia in observational studies. Not surprisingly, this has led to several clinical trials investigating whether postmenopausal hormone replacement therapy can potentially delay/avoid cognitive changes and subsequently, the onset of dementia. However, the evidence of these trials has been mixed, with some showing positive effects while others show no or even negative effects. Controversies remain different in most review articles, existing studies and trials showed conflicting result of association of menopause and cognitive changes and dementia. Therefore, we need to do future interventional studies in more personalized approach toward hormone replacement therapy (HRT) use in postmenopausal women, by taking into account the women's genetic status and for dementia risk.

Estrogen protects against apoptosis and neural injury, and enhances various neurotransmitters such as acetylcholine, which is important in memory processing.[7] So deficiency state of the menopause and mild cognitive impairment is common; though other factors and age itself have much influence. Both menopause and aging brain are associated with potential poor cognitive domain although it can be difficult to distinguish between effects of menopause or from environmental actors.[8,9]

The poor cognition is more marked in premature menopause than in natural menopause as there is sudden declination of estrogen in premature menopause. Estrogens are influential in various neural cellular systems, suggesting mechanisms through which the menopausal decline in estrogen could interfere with cognitive functioning. Whether the patterns and rates of change in hormones over the menopause transition predict changes in cognitive function remains a critical question.

■ PRESENTATION

Women with cognitive impairment most commonly have complaints of difficulty in recalling words or numbers, needing memory aids, and forgetting new things. Although memory complaints are common during menopause,[10] longitudinal data regarding the impact of menopausal hormone changes on cognitive function are limited. Only two longitudinal cohort studies have reported, longitudinal cognitive data for women transitioning through menopause, the Kinmen Women-Health Investigation (KIWI)[11] and the Study of Women's Health across the Nation (SWAN).[12] As reviewed by Greendale et al. (2011),[13] both studies observed decrements in cognitive function specifically in perimenopause. The effects were subtle, evidenced by reduced "learning effects" over repeated cognitive assessments rather than by a decline in cognitive performance. Women may not recognize their poor memory or cognitive problems and confuse with menopause symptoms. Again cognitive complaints are not explained by confounding variables, such as vasomotor symptoms, mood, sleep disturbance, etc.[14] So, detail history and assessment is cornerstone to diagnosis of cognitive impairment.

However, women may present with *impaired cognition* includes:
- Memory issue
- Confusion
- Difficulties in focusing
- Decreased attention.

Some cognitive disorders are temporary or reversible and some are permanent or irreversible. So duration of the forgetfulness and other associated symptoms need to be asked. Most women present with mild cognitive impairment during the menopausal transition with the majority reporting worsening verbal memory. This group of women also suffer from increased risk of mood change and depressive episode. But whether menopause triggers this brain fog or impaired cognition is still a matter of controversy.

Everyone's brain functions change as they age; for most, thought processes, analysis and problem solving show a decline during midlife and beyond.[3] This is because these tasks are linked directly to memory and other mental abilities. When these abilities are affected, women experience symptoms of poor memory, poor concentration, fuzzy thinking or have trouble in multitasking.

The most severe form of cognitive deterioration is dementia.

Dementia

It is primary and progressive irreversible disease. Alzheimer's disease is the most prevalent dementia. There are many risk actors for dementia but old age and female gender are important risk factors for dementia. Dementia severely impacts individuals, and it is no longer possible to carry out normal day-to-day activities. Genetic causes, cholinergic hypothesis, and brain atrophy are the etiology behind. Menopause is not the direct cause of dementia so it is unlikely that menopause lady will represent dementia. If woman comes with dementia, she should not be taken just because of menopause or age related. Age-related cognitive decline on the other hand is not due to the same processes. Age related or in menopause patients can become a little more forgetful and a little less efficient in thinking. Therefore women complaining of severe forgetfulness they need to be referred to the specialists to rule out dementia. The good news is that many aspects of healthy aging of menopause women are under their control. Importantly, healthy aging also provides a buffer against dementia changes that might emerge later in life. Therefore menopause is the time to adopt all the possible strategies to maintain healthy lifestyle, which keeps the brain active and functioning. So when women attend with complains of forgetfulness gynecologists need to assess for poor cognition as well as dementia. Age and the following important determinant factors need to be addressed so that appropriate diagnosis can be made. Early diagnosis and early intervention of dementia may prevent or slow the

progression of disease. Menopause specialists should have idea about mild impaired cognition (MIC), dementia and Alzheimer's disease and their risk factors such as:
- Genetic predisposition
- Busy work
- Depression
- Insomnia
- Stressful life events
- Inadequate social support
- Multiple role player
- Elevated body mass index
- Current smoker status
- African American
- Cardiovascular disease
- Hypertension, diabetes
- Premature menopause
- Job stress
- Anxiety.

Women should aware of symptoms that may be signs of more serious memory problems, such as:
- Repeating questions or comments
- Neglecting hygiene
- Forgetting how to use common objects
- Being unable to understand or follow directions
- Forgetting common words
- Getting lost in places you know well
- Having trouble carrying out basic daily activities.

Experiencing such symptoms, women must attend to specialists so that Alzheimer's disease or dementia can be excluded.

In Alzheimer's disease, the brain shrinks and weighs about two-thirds of its original weight and is characterized by *4 As:*
1. *Agnosia*: Inability to recognize people and objects.
2. *Aphasia*: Language disturbance.
3. *Amentia*: Inability to learn and recall.
4. *Apraxia*: Motor dysfunction. So assessment of these clinical factors are also important, if so detail evaluation is necessary as natural menopause is unlikely the sole reason.

Memory problems are predominantly a function of stressful life and for multiple burdens, which again resulting in diminished attention and concentration.

Premature ovarian insufficiency (POI) or menopause has long-term negative effects on cognitive function and on verbal fluency, memory task

and decline psychomotor speed. Decline of memory is usually most pronounced within 12 months of final menstruation. Premature menopause is menopause before 40 years of age, which can be due to variety of causes:
- Surgery (BSO)
- Chemotherapy
- Radiotherapy
- Chromosomal or genetic defects
- Spontaneous premature ovarian failure.

In contrast to natural menopause, administration of estrogen in POI improves the episodic memory and cognitive function significantly. Usually premature menopause is associated with sharp decline of estrogen, so the short-term cognitive capacity can be improved by estrogen replacement therapy as estrogen does work by enhancing formation of synapses, neurite growth, hippocampus and precotex neurogenesis. Also estrogen therapy protect against apoptosis and neural injury including toxicity induced by excitatory neurotransmitter, amyloid, oxidative stress and ischemia.

■ DIAGNOSIS

Detailed history is the cornerstone, actually we need to diagnose as most menopause women come to us with great hope. Proper diagnosis of mild cognitive impairment MCI, or dementia or Alzheimer's disease gives real justice to the patient. We may follow the American Academy of Neurology (AAN) criteria for diagnosis of memory complains:
- Objective memory impairment
- Normal general thinking and reasoning skill
- Ability to perform normal daily activities.

Sometimes history needs to be taken from the family members. Special attention should be given to medical history (DM, CVS, endocrine, neurology) and drug history of analgesics, sedatives, hypnotics, psychotropics and anticholinergics.

Laboratory investigations need TSH, CBC, RBS, Prolactin, VDRL, Vitamin B_{12} tests to be done and CT scan brain.

■ TREATMENT

It needs to involve multidisciplinary approach, including the participation of menopause specialist, neurologist, geriatric psychiatrist, and mental health specialists.

Menopause is inevitable for all women; the focus should lie with lessening its effects and improving quality-of-life. The risk of memory loss increases after menopause. Many factors can contribute to memory loss but simple lifestyle changes may help prevent the effects of aging and maintain brain health and alertness. Sleep loss contributes to mood disturbances and brain

activities, and leads to depression. Women should maintain a healthy sleep cycle by:
- Maintaining a regular sleep schedule, including on the weekends
- Reducing caffeine intake
- Keeping bedroom cool, and consider placing a fan nearby
- Purchasing a cooling pad or pillows with cooling elements
- Making sure the bedroom is as dark as possible
- Learning relaxation techniques, such as mindful meditation or yoga
- Exercising, but not right before bedtime
- Wearing bedclothes made of natural fibers, such as cotton, hemp, linen, or silk
- Avoiding alcohol, smoking, and spicy foods
- Considering consultation with specialist to arrange a sleep assessment.

Though some women notice forgetfulness or slight cognitive symptoms, which can raise concerns of mental decline, counseling is very important for women who do not have any neurological deficits, they need to be informed that during the menopause transition, there may in fact be modest reductions in aspects of attention[15] but natural menopause does not appear to lead to persistently poorer memory.[16]

There is no definitive list of actions to help reduce memory loss but evidence does support some approaches over others may have roles.[17] Brain health can be improved through mentally stimulating activities, such as work or leisure.[18] Here we will discuss measures of how brain health and functions can be improved.

■ NUTRITION, DIET AND LIFESTYLE MEASURES
Mediterranean Diet

Research suggests that a Mediterranean diet in midlife and beyond supplemented with olive oil or nuts can help improve brain function. It may be the antioxidant-rich diet that is strongly associated with delaying cognitive decline.[19] Orange juice and fresh green vegetables contain more antioxidants. Coffee may stimulate brain activities. But too much coffee is detrimental.

Mediterranean diet is not a specific diet per se more of a lifestyle whereby individuals eat natural, unprocessed foods such as fruits, vegetables, whole grains and nuts. They make olive oil as their primary source of dietary fat; reduce red meat consumption and eating low to moderate amounts of fish.

Diet low in saturated fats, high in omega-3 and rich in antioxidants, whole egg, and chicken are helpful. Coffee seems to protect the brain against cognitive impairments and boost thinking skill. Orange drink reduces the risk of dementia and 34% reduction in memory loss.

Physical Activity

Some studies suggest that physical activity combined with mental stimulation help improve brain health in older adults.[20] Postmenopausal women can also be prone to additional weight gain due to reduced estrogen lowering the metabolic rate so regular exercise will help combat a multitude of symptoms. Although women frequently report weight gain during this period, studies have consistently shown that weight gain is primarily influenced by age, not menopause.[21,22]

Tai chi exercises have proven effective in trials at boosting memory.[23,24] These specific exercises focus one's attention on the here and now, and promote mindfulness; this is an important component of meditation and mind-body practices such as tai chi. Brain also needs some exercise. Keeping brain active helps stave off the effects of aging. Women need to follow these tips to give brain a workout:
- Do crossword, puzzles and Sudoku
- Play word games
- Play online brain games and quizzes
- Read books, newspapers, and magazines
- Learn something new, such as a musical instrument or a new language
- Spend time talking and socializing with family or friends.

Alcohol and Smoking

The studies suggest *reduction of toxins,* including alcohol and smoking, as well as the implementation of mental and physical exercises can prevent cognitive decline in the elderly menopause women.[25] Women in midlife and beyond are advised to have no more than two units of alcohol per day.[26] *Mental activation and social interaction* are very important steps to keep brain active. Mental stimulation such as playing chess and other board games, learning a foreign language, volunteering, reading and playing a musical instrument all keep the brain tuned increasing its capacity and improving cognitive functions.[27-29] Finding a friend to do some of these activities which is also a bonus: in a study that examined over 1,000 people, those with a limited social network were 60% more likely to have cognitive decline and dementia after a three-year period.[30] Socialization, gardening, playing musical instruments or singing and solving puzzles boost up neuronal activities.

Lifestyle Modification

Sleep and enough rest improve cognitive capacity and reduce the level of stress hormone.

Mental activities, recreation tend to improve cognitive capacity. Reading books, singing, gardening, swimming, playing musical instrument, solving puzzles prevent decline in cognition and dementia.

Exercise has been shown to prevent the pathology of AD in high-risk women, meditation helps to relax so meditation should be advised.

Strengthening brain by trying to learn something new one, reading daily keeps the brain functioning and young.

Control of DM, hypertension and menopausal symptoms may be useful in preventing cognitive impairment.

Psychotherapy

Several form of psychotherapy may be helpful including cognitive behavioral therapy (CBT), interpersonal therapy and psychodynamic psychotherapy.

Pharmacotherapy

Menopausal Hormone Therapy

Menopausal hormone therapy (MHT) may not directly impact or improve memory; however, the benefits of this prescribed treatment help to alleviate menopausal symptoms and reduce risk for other diseases in post menopause women. Vasomotor upset, palpitation, feeling of loneliness and dyspareunia have negative effects on mental health, which also contributes poor cognitive capacity. Therefore amelioration of these symptoms may help in some extent to prevent poor cognition. But women need to be discussed that MHT is not the treatment of poor cognition rather it may help other menopausal symptoms. A woman's informed decision is increasingly the critical factor in whether MHT is prescribed for other symptoms if she has and if it is decided right choice for her, by the healthcare professional.[31]

Though estrogen is neurotropic and neuroprotective, affecting serotonergic, cholinergic and dopaminergic systems of brain which are important for cognition and mood. But estrogen therapy during menopause may not improve cognitive function. Rather if MHT initiated in an elderly woman, there is increase the risk of dementia. A critical determinant of the effect of estrogen on CNS and CVS appears to be the timing of estrogen exposure in relation to menopausal transition—that is exposure early in the menopausal transition or postmenopausal period confers cognitive benefit, whereas exposure later in the post menopause confers neutral or detrimental effect (Critical Timing Hypothesis or Healthy Cell Bias Hypothesis). Although the Women's Health Initiative (WHI)/The Women's Health Initiative Memory Study (WHIMS) trials reflected cognitive harm following use of exogenous hormone treatment, since a number of confounds in study design have been identified. Large clinical trials, such as KEEPS-Cog and ELITE, have shown neither deleterious nor beneficial cognitive outcomes with hormone therapy when women are metabolically healthy and treatment commences at or shortly after the menopausal transition. A number of questions regarding hormone therapy remain, particularly the optimal duration of hormone therapy administration and pharmacogenomics interactions related to treatment. To our knowledge, no studies have attempted to fully mimic the premenopausal hormone cycles with menopausal HT, effectively delaying the transition or attenuating the abruptness of change. Data from such a trial would clarify why women's risk for cardiovascular disease shifts upward with menopause, and why women evidence differential risk for AD dementia compared to men.

Selective estrogen receptor modulators (SERM): Tamoxifen used in breast cancer prevention and Raloxifene used in osteoporosis prevention. In large clinical trial, Raloxifene has no effect on overall cognitive function, but Tamoxifen might impair cognitive function. Cognitive effect of SERMs is yet to be studied.

NICE guidelines 2015 focused on the use of MHT for up to 5 years for the symptomatic relief and prevention of progression of chronic diseases.

Antidepressant

Selective serotonin reuptake inhibitor (SSRI)/selective serotonin norepinephrine reuptake inhibitor (SSNRI)—may be helpful to improve cognition if associated with depression.

Acetylcholinesterase Inhibitor

It could be beneficial for patient with early dementia.

■ KEY MESSAGES

- Getting elder and going through menopause does not mean that women will feel old and will have memory problems or dementia.
- Menopause may be associated with mild cognitive impairment, which could be prevented by healthy aging.
- Lifestyle modification, psychotherapy, and MHT in special occasion may prevent cognitive impairment.
- Menopause women complaining memory loss need full evaluation and need exclusion of dementia.
- If cognitive decline is diagnosed, multidisciplinary approach is essential to achieve optimum outcome.
- Menopausal hormone therapy will not induce cognitive harm, it is supported by the recent and large controlled trials specifically when treatment is initiated at or near the menopausal transition or at the time of oophorectomy may provide short-term cognitive benefits.
- Menopause-related cognitive issues "need not compromise a woman's quality-of-life," though women may have to be proactive for the condition to be properly diagnosed and treated.
- Having mental recreation, social engagement, playing puzzles, learning new languages, mixing with friends keep the brain active and delays degeneration.

REFERENCES

1. Sharman S. Defining the menopausal transition. Am J Med. 2005;118:3-7.
2. Sliwinski JR, Johnson AK, Elkins GR. Memory decline in peri- and post-menopausal women: the potential of mind-body medicine to improve cognitive performance integrative medicine. Insights. 2014:9;17-23.
3. Burger HG, Cahir N, Robertson DM, Groome NP, Dudley E, Green AL, et al. Serum inhibins A and B fall differentially as FSH rises in perimenopausal women. Clin Endocrinol. 1998;48:809-13.
4. McEwen B. Estrogen actions throughout the brain. Recent Prog Horm Res. 2002;57:357-384.
5. Henderson VW. Cognitive changes after menopause: influence of estrogen clinical obstetrics gynecology. Clin Obstet Gynecol. 2008;51:618-26.
6. Greendale GA, Derby CA, Maki PM. Perimenopause and cognition. Obstet Gynecol Clin North Am. 2011;38:519-35.
7. Craig MC, Fletcher PC, Daly EM, Rymer J, Brammer M, Giampietro V, et al. The interactive effect of the cholinergic system and acute ovarian suppression on the brain: an fMRI study. Horm Behav. 2009;55:41-9.
8. Will MA, Randolph JF. The influence of reproductive hormones on brain function in the menopausal transition. Minerva Ginecol. 2009;61:469-81.
9. Henderson VW, Popat RA. Effects of endogenous and exogenous estrogen exposures in midlife and late-life women on episodic memory and executive functions. Neuroscience. 2011;191:129-38.
10. Sullivan Mitchell E, Fugate Woods N. Midlife women's attributions about perceived memory changes: observations from the Seattle Midlife Women's Health Study. J Womens Health Gend Based Med. 2001;10:351-62.
11. Fuh JL, Wang SJ, Lee SJ, Lu SR, Juang KD. A longitudinal study of cognition change during early menopausal transition in a rural community. Maturitas. 2006;53:447-53.
12. Greendale GA, Huang MH, Wight RG, Seeman T, Luetters C, Avis NE, et al. Effects of the menopause transition and hormone use on cognitive performance in midlife women. Neurology. 2009;72:1850-7.
13. Greendale GA, Derby CA, Maki PM. Perimenopause and cognition. Obstet Gynecol Clin North Am. 2011;38:519-35.
14. Greendale GA, Wight RG, Huang MH, Avis N, Gold EB, Joffe H, et al. Menopause-associated symptoms and cognitive performance: results from the study of women's health across the nation. Am J Epidemiol. 2010;171:1214-24.
15. Weber MT, Mapstone M, Staskiewicz J, Maki PM. Reconciling subjective memory complaints with objective memory performance in the menopausal transition. Menopause. 2012;19:735-41.
16. Henderson VW. Gonadal hormones and cognitive aging: a midlife perspective. Womens Health (Lond). 2011;7:81-93.
17. Williams JW, Plassman BL, Burke J, Holsinger T, Benjamin S. Preventing Alzheimer's Disease and Cognitive Decline. Evidence Report/Technology Assessment Number 193. Department of Health and Human Services. Rockville, MD: Agency for Healthcare Research and Quality; 2010.
18. Henderson VW. Three midlife strategies to prevent cognitive impairment due to Alzheimer's disease. Climacteric. 2014;17(2):38-46.
19. Valls-Pedret C, Sala-Vila A, Serra-Mir M, Corella D, de la Torre R, Martínez-González MÁ, et al. Mediterranean diet and age-related cognitive decline: a randomized clinical trial. JAMA Intern Med. 2015;175(7):1094-103.
20. Rahe J, Petrelli A, Kaesberg S, Fink GR, Kessler J, Kalbe E. Effects of cognitive training with additional physical activity compared to pure cognitive training in healthy older adults. Clin Interv Aging. 2015;10:297-310.

21. Sternfeld B, Wang H, Quesenberry CP Jr, Abrams B, Everson-Rose SA, Greendale GA, et al. Physical activity and changes in weight and waist circumference in midlife women: findings from the Study of Women's Health Across the Nation. Am J Epidemiol. 2004;160:912-22.
22. Guthrie JR, Dennerstein L, Dudley EC. Weight gain and the menopause: a 5-year prospective study. Climacteric. 1999;2:205-11.
23. Taylor-Piliae RE, Newell KA, Cherin R, Lee M, King AC, Haskell WL. Tai Chi versus Western exercise on physical and cognitive functioning in healthy community-dwelling older adults: a randomized clinical trial. J Aging Phys Act. 2010;18:261-79.
24. Mortimer JA, Ding D, Borenstein AR, DeCarli C, Guo Q, Wu Y, et al. Changes in brain volume and cognition in a randomized trial of exercise and social interaction in a community-based sample of non-demented Chinese elders. J Alzheimers Dis. 2012;30:757-66.
25. Williams JW, Plassman BL, Burke J, Holsinger T, Benjamin S. Preventing Alzheimer's Disease and Cognitive Decline. Evidence Report/Technology Assessment Number 193. Rockville: Agency for Healthcare Research and Quality; 2010.
26. Wikipedia. Recommended maximum intake of alcoholic beverages. [online] Available from: en.wikipedia.org/wiki/Recommended_maximum_intake_of_alcoholic_beverages. [Last accessed March, 2021].
27. Henderson VW. Three midlife strategies to prevent cognitive impairment due to Alzheimer's disease. Climacteric. 2014;17(Suppl 2):38-46.
28. Stern Y. Cognitive reserve in aging and Alzheimer's disease. Lancet Neurology 2012;11.
29. Reijnders J, van Heugten C, van Boxtel M. Cognitive interventions in healthy older adults and people with mild cognitive impairment: a systematic review. Ageing Res Rev. 2013;12:263-75.
30. Friedman Richard A. Forget Something? Then Read This. New York Times. 2007.
31. Manson JE, Chlebowski RT, Stefanick ML, Aragaki AK, Rossouw JE, Prentice RL, et al. Menopausal hormone therapy and health outcomes during the intervention and extended post stopping phases of the Women's Health Initiative randomized trials. JAMA. 2013;310:1353-68.

CHAPTER 9

Sexuality and Menopause

■ INTRODUCTION

There is marked decline in all the domains of sexual function such as desire, arousal, orgasm and pain in both women and men, as they grow older. The androgen milieu and sexual desire seem to be tightly linked so both decline with age. Menopause is milestone in women's life; withdrawal of hormone estrogen, testosterone, dehydroepiandrosterone (DEHA) exacerbates the female sexual dysfunction (FSD) more than men.[1] Menopause happens so dramatically that women feel a great challenge to cope with that than their counterpart. But sexual well-being of menopausal women depends not only on menopause or hormone deficiency. Hormone deficiency is one of the factors but social, cultural and psychological and personal issues, which grouped into *Biopsychosocial model*. The Biopsychosocial model has tremendous role on female sexuality.[2] Biopsychosocial model includes the women's personal attitude toward sex, social belief, religious culture, and relationship with the partner, comorbidities of the partner or herself. Interpersonal relationship is the most important criteria for the sexual well-being for women. Study shows that women place high value on sexual intimacy in their relationship.[3,4] PRESIDE study[5] and Revive study showed that vaginal dryness during menopause adversely affect the enjoyment 72% and women felt sexual spontaneity about 66%.[6] Diminished sexuality of women may break the relationship and women may suffer from severe mental depression. But irony is, women suffer silently, they do not express or share the problem with anyone. In some community, it is a taboo so many women refrain from sex. On the contrary health providers do not ask this issue or they are unaware of the issue. So the issue of sexuality remains unresolved and keeping the FSD in menopause, difficult to address. Though very few women complain of decreased sexuality but that is actually the tip of the iceberg. While addressing sexuality doctors need to know the latest classification of FSD, which is, classified according to the Diagnostic and Statistical Manual of Mental Disorders, fifth edition (DSM-5):
- Female sexual interest and arousal disorder
- Female sexual orgasmic disorder
- Genito-pelvic pain/penetration disorder
- Substance/medication-induced sexual dysfunction.

The loss of estrogen and testosterone following menopause can lead to changes in a woman›s body and sexual drive. So menopausal or elderly women usually suffer from 1st and 2nd type of sexual dysfunction. They feel less interest in sex. Also, lower levels of estrogen can cause a drop in blood supply to the vagina. That can affect vaginal lubrication, causing the vagina to be too dry for comfortable sex. Women having dry vagina suffer from severe dyspareunia.

The International vaginal health; insight, views, and attitudes (VIVA) study reported the prevalence of specific symptoms including vaginal dryness (83%) and pain during sex (42%).[7] But interestingly some postmenopausal women feel an improved *sex drive*. That may be due to less *anxiety* linked to a fear of *pregnancy*. Also, many postmenopausal women often have fewer child-rearing responsibilities and no more household choirs, allowing them to relax and enjoy *intimacy* with their husbands.

Sexual behavior is controlled by a hormonally response neural network. Endocrine, neurological, psychiatric conditions, cancer medication and surgical procedures, alcohol intake, local diseases, deficient estrogen-testosterone, biopsychosocial factors all these have influence on sexuality. Nothing happens without desire again painful sex affects desire and all other domains of sexual cycle. The decrease in circulating estrogen levels during and after the menopause transition, along with the age-associated decline in androgen, independent of menopause, significantly contribute low desire, poor arousal, dyspareunia, impaired orgasm and consequently reduced sexual satisfaction.[8] In addition, menopause may impact emotional and cognitive aspects of sexuality through personal experiences including age at menopause, type of menopause, physical and mental health, achievement of reproductive goals, education, body image, and self-esteem norms and experience. Psychosocial factors are important factors for sexuality.[9] Also partner issues strongly correlate with FSD and quality-of-life.[10] Nonetheless, it is need to be aware that even not complaining postmenopausal women may also experience sexual concerns and difficulties that need to be addressed.[11,12]

■ DIAGNOSIS

For diagnosis, history taking needs to be very meticulous and empathetic. It should be focusing on her cultural, social, religious belief, personal relationship and comorbidities of the woman and for her husband. Finding the source of the issue is most important to treat the problem. After detailed history taking, clinical examination including per-vaginal examination is necessary so that local pathology can be excluded.

We need to follow The DSM5 guidelines (American Psychiatric Press, USA, 2013) to diagnose female sexual dysfunction even for menopause women. During history taking special consideration should be paid to lack of interest in sex and pain disorder as decreased arousal is common in menopause. Although sexual desire triggers arousal but in menopause, desire will follow arousal, healthcare providers need to keep it in mind while treating them. Lack of orgasm in non-aroused women makes sex less pleasurable. So it is vital for women to be aroused for enjoyable sex. Again withdrawal of hormone makes the vaginal wall very thin friable, less elastic, dry and it becomes prone to mechanical damage during sex. Lack of lubrication needs to be enquired as it causes painful intercourse.

Minimum investigations are done to exclude other causes than menopause for sexual dysfunction.

TREATMENT

Treatment strategies depend on probable cause and type of sexual dysfunction. It may focus on:
- Treating any medical comorbidities
- Providing sex education
- Teaching sexual behavior, response, performances
- Enhancing stimulation
- Use of erotic videos, books, masturbation
- Providing destruction technique
- Use of erotic and nonerotic fantasies, exercises
- Minimizing pain if dyspareunia.

Team approach is important and most of the sexual dysfunctions in menopause women can be solved if underlying physical and psychological causes are corrected.

Multidisciplinary team should include sex therapist, psychologists, gynecologists, and sex counselors. To achieve the best result they need to work together with the holistic approach.

General Treatment

Lifestyle modification with maintenance of optimum body weight is the cornerstone, it has positive impact on sexuality and prevents emergence of new diseases. Daily exercise, avoidance of stress, having mental recreation, and buildup of self-confidence improves the sexual desire and performances in this group of women. Enhancing good relationship with partner and better understanding with the partner are very important factors to improve sexuality. Treatment of all comorbidities of both partners is required for improving the sexual function.

Alternative Therapy

Sex toys and devices may help in arousal in some women. Use of vibrator stimulates clitoris. Sex therapists use clitoral vacuum suction, which is helpful but very expensive. Dilators are also helpful if there is severe vaginal stenosis. Counseling with sex therapists and sex counselors are much effective.

Medical Therapy

Menopause women suffer from hormone deficiency due to estrogen withdrawal, they develop vaginal dryness which results dyspareunia and this single entity of dyspareunia affects all the domain of sexual function. In this case, estrogen is the first choice in vulvovaginal atrophy (VVA) as it ameliorates the dryness and improves dyspareunia. Local application of estrogen can be used at a stretch for 6-12 months. Systemic estrogen therapy does not have much impact to improve the sexual function for menopause women.

Local DHEA, moisturizer, and lubricants are also helpful. Local DHEA cream is very effective treatment for dyspareunia second—dry to VVA but oral DHEA has no significant role.[13,14]

Systemic non-hormonal therapy: Ospemifene is effective (approved by US and EU). Daily oral doses (60 mg/day) of Ospemifene are effective to enhance decreased libido.

Botox is not yet evidence-based but many women may get good result. G-shot is very popular in USA where PRP is injected beneath the vaginal mucosa at the junction of upper one-third and lower two-thirds of mucosa. G-shot may stimulate sexual orgasm, but again it is not yet evidence-based to recommend routinely.

Laser therapy is very promising to correct underlying hypoestrogenic changes of vagina. But it cannot stimulate brain for desire or orgasm. So it is only for local use.

Tibolone: It has androgenic action so in some extent it helps to improve libido. But it's use is limited as there is concern of trigger the recurrence of breast cancer.[15]

Flibanserin (Addyi®), used for increased desire or sex drive (FDA approved) 100 mg dose at bed time, it is centrally acting oral multifunctioning serotonin agonist. About 50-60% women respond to flibanserin. It is safe and effective.[16]

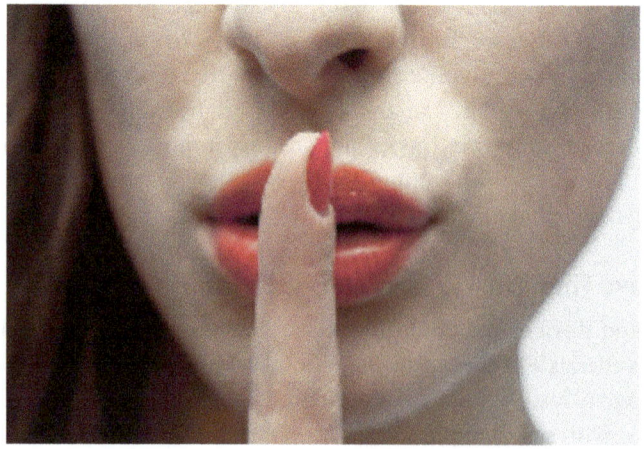

Sildenafil (Viagra) are being used but unlike in men, expected result is not found in women for improving sexual dysfunction.[17]

Testosterone is the key hormone for desire and arousal, so it can be used if there is no contraindication. Hypoactive sexual desire disorder (HSDD), a subset of FSD, causes personal distress for surgically and naturally postmenopausal and premenopausal women. HSDD has a multifactorial etiology, including psychosocial factors such as relationship issues and medical factors such as medications, chronic illnesses, and hormonal effects. Several randomized controlled trials showed significant improvement in the sexual function of premenopausal and naturally and surgically postmenopausal women with testosterone therapy.[18]

Testosterone, administered transdermally as a cream, patch or gel or as an implanted pellet, improves sexual well-being in postmenopausal women with low sexual desire associated distress.[19] 150–300 µg/day of testosterone is recommended for decreased libido. International Menopause Society (IMS) has published Position Paper on testosterone, which clearly mentioned that testosterone can be used in diminished libido for menopause women. It should not be continued beyond 6 months if women do not get any response. Although no androgen therapies for HSDD are available in Canada, the reviewed clinical evidence supports the safety of short-term testosterone therapy for postmenopausal women with HSDD. The evidence we have reviewed here suggests that transdermal testosterone, at a dose of 150 µg or 300 µg per day, appears to be the safest method of administration. The 52-week APHRODITE trial of 814 women found no cases of endometrial hyperplasia or carcinoma.[13] More women using a 300 µg transdermal testosterone patch reported vaginal bleeding (10.6%) than women using a 150 µg patch (2.7%) or placebo (2.6%). However, all women underwent endometrial biopsy, transvaginal ultrasonography, or both, and only two women who were using a 300 µg patch had proliferative endometrium on biopsy.

More long-term studies investigating the safety of testosterone therapy in women are needed.

Bupropion 300–400 mg daily improves sexual interest. It reduces serotonin inhibition. Potential future therapies include bremelanotide and combination of testosterone/sildenafil or testosterone/buspirone (Martha Rosenberg, Center for Health Journalism).

■ KEY MESSAGES
- Positive sexual function at midlife can enhance personal and relationship quality, improve longevity and enhance quality-of-life.
- FSD causes many sufferings to these groups of women; even it breaks the relationship and leaves the women isolated with extreme inferiority complex and with mental agony.

- Self-reporting is rare in our country and history taking is not so simple so health providers need to be proactive and they should possess not only the necessary wide medical knowledge, but also need empathy and compassion for menopause women.
- The loss of estrogen and testosterone following menopause can lead to physiological and emotional changes in a woman's body that can impact on their sex life, including: Painful or uncomfortable sex occurs due to reduced vaginal secretions and thinning of the vagina, women suffer from loss of libido (lower sex drive), higher incidence of *Candida albicans* (thrush) and bacterial vaginosis (BV).
- Body changes that lower self-esteem such as thinning of hair and breast changes.
- Not all women experience problems but for those who do they should be encouraged to discuss their worries with their partners and work together.
- Lubricants and moisturizers, vaginal estrogen creams, menopause hormone therapy (MHT) should be encouraged. Avoidance of precipitants that exacerbates vaginal dryness and increases the incidence of BV and thrush such as vaginal deodorants or tight, restricted clothing.
- Need to promote continence by encouraging pelvic floor exercises or referral to continence services.
- Couple should take time with love making to make women more aroused and explore new ways to enjoy sexual pleasure.
- Multiprofessional team approach may bring the success to enhance sexuality of menopause women.

REFERENCES

1. Lindau ST, Schumm LP, Laumann EO, Levinson W, O'Muircheartaigh CA, Waite LJ. A study of sexuality and health among older adults in the UNITED States. N Engl J Med. 2007;357(8):762-74.
2. Janssen I, Powell LH, Crawford S, Lasley B, Sutton-Tyrrell K. Menopause and the metabolic syndrome: the study of women's health across the nation. Arch Intern Med. 2008;168(14):1568-75.
3. Foodladi E, Bell RJ, Whittaker AM, Davis SR. Women's expectations and experiences of hormone treatment for sexual dysfunction. Climacteric. 2014;17(6):674-81.
4. Tan HM, Marumo K, Yang DY, Hwang TI, Ong ML. Sex among Asian women: the Global Better sex survey in Asia. Int J Urol. 2009;16(5):507-14.
5. Shifren JL, Monz BU, Russo PA, Segreti A, Johannes CB. Sexual problems and distress in United States women; prevalence and correlates. Obstet Gynecol. 2008;112(5):970-8.
6. Nappi RE, Kingsberg S, Maamari R, Simon J. The CLOSER survey: implications of vaginal discomfort in postmenopausal women and in male partners. J Sex Med. 2013;10(9):2232-41.
7. Nappi RE, Kokot-Kierepa M. Vaginal Health: insight, Views and Attitude (VIVA)-results from an international survey. Climacteric. 2012;15(1):36-44..
8. Wåhlin-Jacobsen S, Pedersen AT, Kristensen E, Laessøe NC, Lundqvist M, Cohen AS, et al. Is there a correlation between androgen and sexual desire in women? J Sex Med. 2015;12(2):358-73.

9. Hawton K, Gath D, Day A. Sexual function in a community sample of middle aged women with partners: effects of age, martial, socioeconomic, psychiatric, gynecological and menopausal factors. Arch Sex Behav. 1994;23(4):375-95.
10. Chedraui P, Pérez-López FR, Mezones-Holguin E, San Miguel G, Avila C, Collaborative Group for Research of the Climacteric in Latin America. Assessing predictors of sexual function in mid aged sexually active women. Maturitas. 2011;68(4):387-90.
11. Worsley R, Bell RJ, Gartoulla P, Davis SR. Prevalence and predictors of low sexual desire dysfunction in a community based sample of midlife women. J Sex Med. 2017;14(5):675-86.
12. Zelek BM, Bell RJ, Billah B, Davis SR. Hypoactive sexual desire dysfunction in community dwelling older women. Menopause. 2017;24(4):391-9.
13. Alkatib AA, Cosma M, Elamin MB, Erickson D, Swiglo BA, Erwin PJ, et al. A systemic review and meta-analysis of randomized placebo controlled trial of DHEA treatment effects on quality of life in women with adrenal insufficiency. J Clin Endocrinol Metab. 2009;94(10):3676-81.
14. Elraiyah T, Sonbol MB, Wang Z, Khairalseed T, Asi N, Undavalli C, et al. Clinical review: the benefits and harms of systemic DHEA in postmenopausal women with normal adrenal function: a systemic review and meta-analysis. J Clin Endocrinol Metab. 2014;99(10):3536-42.
15. Henderson VW. Alzheimer's disease: review of hormone therapy trials and implications for treatment and prevention after menopause. J Steroid Biochem Mol Biol. 2014;142:99-106.
16. Katz M, DeRogatis LR, Ackerman R, Hedges P, Lesko L, Garcia M Jr, et al. Efficacy of flibanserin in women with hypoactive sexual desire disorder: results from the BEGONIA trial. J Sex Med. 2013;10(7):1807-15.
17. NEJM Journal Watch. Women's Health. [online] Available from: https://www.jwatch.org/womens-health [Last accessed March, 2021].
18. Panay N, Al-Azzawi F, Bouchard C, Davis S, Eden J, Lodhi I, et al. Testosterone treatment of HSDD in naturally menopausal women: the ADORE study. Climacteric. 2010;13:121-31.
19. Wierman ME, Arlt W, Basson R, Davis SR, Miller KK, Murad MH, et al. Androgen therapy in women; a reappraisal; an endocrine society clinical practice guideline. J Clin Endocrinol Metab. 2014;99(10):3489-510.

CHAPTER 10

Contraceptives in Perimenopause

■ INTRODUCTION

While perimenopausal women have low fecundity, they are still capable of becoming pregnant. The unintended pregnancies of this age are associated with more complications such as diabetes, hypertension, miscarriage, baby with congenital anomalies and psychosocial disorders. However, many women and healthcare providers believe that older women should not take oral and other contraceptives because doing so may be dangerous. But unintended pregnancy pushes women toward huge medical problems with life risk and psychosocial embarrassment. Contraception remains important during perimenopause, as women cannot be certain of infertility until they reach 1 year postmenopause. The menopause ranges from 45 to 52 years in most country, 51 in Australia.[1] The pregnancy rate in women 45–49 years is 2–3%, and 1% after age 50 years. About 50% pregnancies in USA are unintended, which includes perimenopausal women.[2]

Australian study suggests that conception is <1 per 100 in women aged >50 years.[3] Abortion occurs in one-fourth of pregnancies in women aged >40 years.[4]

Therefore, women in perimenopause should have access to full array of options of contraceptives to prevent unintended pregnancy hence the complications.

■ OPTIONS OF CONTRACEPTIVES

Contraceptive choice depends on several factors, including medical eligibility, side effects, and gynecological problems. The UK Medical Eligibility Criteria (UKMEC) and Centers for Disease Control and Prevention (CDC) made frameworks for prescribing contraceptives.

All contraceptives are potentially suitable and none is contraindicated by age alone, but use of combined oral contraceptives (COCs), the vaginal ring and depot-medroxyprogesterone acetate (DMPA) are not recommended in those aged >50.[5]

Women aged ≥40 years have an increased risk of comorbidities such as diabetes, high blood pressure. Meticulous history taking, considering climacteric symptoms, and clinical assessments are important factors to take into account to prescribe contraceptives. Contraceptives options are:
- Combined oral contraceptives (COCs) estrogen and progesterone combination
- Progestogen-only methods

- Intrauterine contraceptive devices (IUCD)
- Barrier method
- Nonhormonal methods
- Tubal ligations.

Combined Oral Contraceptives

These offer various health benefits beside contraceptive benefits,[6] which improve quality-of-life. Unfortunately women believe that they should not take COCs because it may be dangerous.[7]

Even physicians are reluctant to prescribe estrogen in fear of increased risks for breast cancer, cardiovascular disease, and venous thromboembolism (VTE)[8] for these group of women.

CDC do not list age itself as a contraindication for COC. Combined pills may cause shorter withdrawal and unscheduled bleeding; in such situation, tailored regimens with prolonged pill-taking or shorter pill-free intervals are effective, reliable and safe.[9]

CDC presented guidelines regarding contraceptive use in women with medical conditions[10] only age restriction of COCs is for women aged 35 years or older who smoke (15 or more cigarettes per day).[10]

One study found risk of cervical cancer 10% increased less than 5 years of use, 60% increased risk with 5-9 years of use;[11] however, the risk declines over time after women stop COC, more evidences are required to confirm it.

COCs that contain certain third-generation progestins (gestodene and desogestrel) may be more thrombophilic than those containing first- or second-generation progestins.

COC containing levonorgestrel, norethisterone and norgestimate having the lowest risk.[12] Unanimous results suggest that there is not statistically significant association between the use of progestogen-only pills (POPs) and VTE.[13]

Women aged 40 years or older can use COCs if they are not obese, non-smokers, have normal blood pressure, and do not have any cardiovascular disease or risk factors[14] and women >44 years should continue contraception if they do not want to become pregnant.[15]

COCs are a highly effective contraceptive method, with a failure rate of <1%.[16] Unfortunately COCs use among perimenopause women is lower than youngster.[17] Its main concerns are:

- *Thromboembolism*:
  - The relative risk for VTE with third-generation versus second-generation progestins is 1.3 (95% CI 1.0-1.8).
  - Decreasing estrogen in COCs resulted slight decrease in the risk of VTE.[18] The incidence of VTE is less (1/7) in Korea than (1/8) in Denmark.[19] Drospirenone has antimineralocorticoid properties, systematic review suggests, drospirenone-containing OCP use is

associated with a higher risk for VTE than both no oral contraceptive pill (OCP) and levonorgestrel-containing OCP use.[20]
- The highest quality studies suggest there are no or slightly increased harmful effects of drospirenone, but their confidence limits do not rule out the risk.[21]
- A large international prospective observational study showed no increased risk for VTE among women taking COCs with drospirenone.[22] However, the increase risk of VTE with COC is 1/10, which is less than ½ that happens in pregnancy.[23] Most COCs will improve acne.[24] Risk factors of VTE are major surgery, thrombophilia, history of VTE/pulmonary embolism, etc.[25]
- Therefore, when recommending COC, detailed history taking with risk assessment is most important. Similarly women should be informed about the risks, so women can accurately understand the impact of COCs and can take decision.[26]

- *Myocardial infarction (MI)*: Combined oral contraceptives increase the relative risk of MI by 1.6-fold, when this risk is applied to the MI incidence among Korean women aged 45–54 years (9.6 per 10,000 persons).[27] The additional incidence of MI due to taking COCs was 5.7 per 10,000/year, which is rare event.
- *Breast cancer*:
  - This is most complex issue and studies, mostly done before the year 2000, suggested that COCs increase risk of breast cancer.[28]
  - Recent studies reported that the risk of breast cancer of COCs with lower estrogen is lower than previously reported (RR = 1.08).[29]
  - Combined oral contraceptive users have a small increased risk of developing breast cancer [odds ratio (OR) 1.5] compared with nonusers[30] but risks decrease after cessation. COC use does not increase overall cancer risks and does not increase cancer mortality risk.[31] Rather COC is protective against ovarian, endometrial and colorectal cancer.
  - Women aged 40 or older can safely use COCs if they are not obese, non-smokers, and do not have any cardiovascular risk factors.[32]

Progestogen-only Methods

Progestogen pill is more effective for women aged >40 years than for women who are younger. However, it may cause poor cycle control, may require investigation to exclude pathology. POPs do not raise blood pressure or alters blood pressure, and POPs do not increased venous risk.[33]

It is effective alternative to COC for comorbidities: The low progestogen dose has very few contraindications.

A levonorgestrel intrauterine device (LNG-IUD) provides 5 years of effective contraception and can be kept until menopause. It reduces menstrual bleeding, thereby ameliorates the abnormal uterine bleeding (AUB) and has few contraindications such as breast cancer.

The Faculty of Sexual and Reproductive Healthcare (FSRH) guidance supports (LNG-IUD) use in women >45 years up to 7 years, or up to menopause.[34]

Depot-medroxyprogesterone Acetate

Depot-medroxyprogesterone acetate is not recommended as first-line management in women aged >45 years and beyond 50 years because it slightly reduces bone density and alters lipids.

The FSRH states, POPs outweigh the benefits in women with multiple risk factors for cardiovascular disease.[35]

Contraceptive Implant

The etonogestrel implant can be used until menopause and has few contraindications (breast cancer), it is associated with minimum metabolic effects and no reduction in bone density.

However, it is associated with prolonged or frequent bleeding. This can mask other causes of irregular bleeding such as endometrial cancer, although this is rare in perimenopause but evaluation is needed.[36]

They are safe in women who smoke and having migraine over 35 years.[37]

Copper Intrauterine Device

The copper IUD is the oldest non-hormonal method for 10 years. It is contraindicated in menorrhagia, uterine fibroids, or previous cervical surgery and have minimal systemic effects so can be safely used in women with comorbidities.

The contraceptive efficacy of the 2nd (Multiload Cu-250 and Nova-T) and 3rd generation (T Cu-380A and Multiload Cu-375) IUDs is higher than older copper IUDs. IUD is associated with a small risk of pelvic inflammatory diseases (PID) in first 20 days after insertion, which suggests that not IUD rather inadequate aseptic technique during insertion of IUD is responsible for the infection.[38]

Moreover studies have suggested that the risk of PID is related more to lifestyle of the user rather than to the device itself.[39]

Barrier Methods

Both male and female condoms prevent sexually transmissible infections and contraception. But compliance is very important.

Sterilization

Female sterilization is a permanent and highly successful form of contraceptive. All women considering sterilization must be counseled regarding long-acting reversible contraception (LARC) methods, as they will shortly reach menopause. Anyway women need to use another method until 3 months passes after the procedure.

Natural Methods

Perimenopausal patients should be advised that these methods are made more difficult and unreliable because of the increasingly irregular menstrual cycles at this stage.

Emergency Contraception

Oral emergency contraception (EC) includes a 1.5 mg levonorgestrel dose, licensed up to 72 hours after unprotected sex, but is effective up to 96 hours.[40]

The newer ulipristal acetate (UPA) appears to have superior efficacy, and is licensed up to 120 hours after unprotected sex. The Cu-IUD (within 5 days of unprotected sex) provides very effective EC and can be used as an on-going long-term method.[41]

Future Development

Ulipristal acetate, a selective progesterone receptor modulator currently licensed as an EC, which will provide effective estrogen free contraception. But UPA may cause endometrial thickening, glandular cystic dilation and unscheduled heavy bleeding.[42]

Frameless IUD consisting of 20 tiny copper spheres of greater potential for the use in nonuniform endometrial cavities.[43]

■ BENEFITS OF CONTRACEPTION

Approximately 90% of women AUB for the 4–8 years before menopause is reached. Once other underlying causes are eliminated, menstrual cycles can be effectively controlled by using COCs in 80% of cases.[44]

Menorrhagia is reduced >50% among 70% of those taking, estradiol/dienogest combination can reduce so estradiol valerate/dienogest (E_2V/DNG) is highly effective for the treatment of AUB.[45] COCs also reduce dysmenorrhea, for which continuous regimen is required.[46] It may also help in vasomotor symptoms.[47]

Women taking COCs for at least 6 years prior to menopause can significantly increase postmenopausal bone mass density as compared to those not taking COC.[48]

COCs also have a preventive effect for some diseases. COCs reduce the risk of endometrial cancer, and this effect appears immediately after administration and increases proportionately with the duration of use. Even after the drug is discontinued, the effect can be sustained for 30 years.[5] A preventive effect, against epithelial ovarian cancer also appears within the first year of drug administration, increases proportionately with duration of use, and is sustained for 20-30 years after discontinuation. Even if the duration of drug administration is less than 1 year, the risk reduction effect can be sustained for 20 years after discontinuation.[6,7] Use of COCs can also reduce colorectal cancer by approximately 20%.[8] As the incidence of cancer increases with age, the preventive effect of COCs on cancer can be considered especially important for middle-aged women. COCs also have bone protection effects. After the age of 40 years, bone mineral density (BMD) is known to decrease by 1% each year.

Women taking COCs for at least 6 years prior to menopause can significantly increase postmenopausal BMD in the femur neck and lumbar spine, as compared to those not taking COC.[45] COCs can also aid in reducing the risk of endometrial cancer, ovarian cancer, and colorectal cancer, as well as maintaining BMD.

Recommendations from the American Society for Reproductive Medicine and North American Menopause Society indicate that contraceptives need to be used 1 year after menopause.[49]

American College of Obstetricians and Gynecologists states regular screening of mammography every 1-2 years between ages 40 and 50; thereafter, it should be performed annually.[50]

Hormone therapy does not provide adequate contraception. Clinicians should carefully consider the associated risks while prescribing contraceptive advice to perimenopausal women. To maximize long-term health in perimenopausal women, clinicians should address smoking cessation, cancer screening, cholesterol screening, and bone loss prevention measures.

■ KEY MESSAGES

- No accurate biological marker exists that truly defines when fertility ceases. Furthermore, pregnancy in older women is associated with increased complications such as miscarriage, high blood pressure, diabetes and chromosomal anomalies with the baby.
- Therefore, perimenopausal women must use contraception to avoid unintended pregnancies therefore, avoiding psychosocial and potential domestic consequences.
- The annual risk of death of woman, associated with using no use of contraceptives exceeds far that for use of any methods among women of all ages.
- No method of contraception is contraindicated for women <50 years on the basis of age alone.
- Menopausal hormone therapy (MHT) does not provide adequate contraception and COC provides non-contraceptive benefits. After taking a comprehensive medical history and assessing risk factors, counseling should be done for risks and benefits.
- It remains a critical aspect in empowering women to make informed choices.

- For users of both hormonal and non-hormonal methods, the time at which it is discontinuing provides an opportunity to discuss the risks and benefits of MHT for the management of the menopause.

REFERENCES

1. Morabia A, Costanza MC. International variability in ages at menarche, first livebirth, and menopause. World Health Organization Collaborative Study of Neoplasia and Steroid Contraceptives. Am J Epidemiol. 1998;148(12):1195-205.
2. Finer LB, Zolna MR. Unintended pregnancy in the United States: incidence and disparities, 2006. Contraception. 2011;84:478-85.
3. Trussell J, Wilson C. Sterility in a population with natural fertility. Population Studies. 2010;39(2):269-86.
4. Scheil W, Scott J, Catcheside B. Pregnancy outcome in South Australia 2014. Adelaide: SA Health Pregnancy Outcome Unit; 2016.
5. Faculty of Sexual and Reproductive Healthcare. Progestogen-only injectable contraception. London: Faculty of Sexual and Reproductive Healthcare; 2014.
6. Lurie G, Wilkens LR, Thompson PJ, McDuffie KE, Carney ME, Terada KY, et al. Combined oral contraceptive use and epithelial ovarian cancer risk: time-related effects. Epidemiology. 2008;19:237-43.
7. Linton A, Golobof A, Shulman LP. Contraception for the perimenopausal woman. Climacteric. 2016;19:526-34.
8. Cho MK. Use of Combined Oral Contraceptives in Perimenopausal Women. Chonnam Med J. 2018;54(3):153-8.
9. Faculty of Sexual and Reproductive Healthcare of the Royal College of Obstetricians and Gynaecologists. FSRH clinical guidance: combined hormonal contraception. London: FSRH; 2012.
10. Curtis KM, Tepper NK, Jatlaoui TC, Berry-Bibee E, Horton LG, Zapata LB, et al. US Medical Eligibility Criteria for Contraceptive Use, 2016. MMWR Recomm Rep. 2016;65:1-103.
11. Smith JS, Green J, Berrington de Gonzalez A, Appleby P, Peto J, Plummer M, et al. Cervical cancer and use of hormonal contraceptives: a systematic review. Lancet. 2003;361(9364):1159-67.
12. Stegeman B, de Bastos M, Rosendaal FR, van Hylckama Vileg A, Helmerhorst FM, Stijnen T, et al. Different combined oral contraceptives and the risk of venous thrombosis: systematic review and network meta-analysis. BMJ. 2013;347:f5298.
13. Lidegaard O, Lokkegaard E, Svendsen AL, Agger C. Hormonal contraception and risk of venous thromboembolism: national follow-up study. BMJ. 2009;339:b2890.
14. Mendoza N, Soto E, Sánchez-Borrego R. Do women aged over 40 need different counseling on combined hormonal contraception? Maturitas. 2016;87:79-83.
15. Curtis KM, Jatlaoui TC, Tepper NK, Zapata LB, Horton LG, Jamieson DJ, et al. US Selected Practice Recommendations for contraceptive Use, 2016. MMWR Recomm Rep. 2016;65:1-66.
16. Trussell J. Contraceptive technology. In: Hatcher RA, Trussell J, Nelson AL, Cates W, Kwal D, Policar MS (Eds). Contraceptive efficacy, 20th edition. New York: Ardent Media; 2011. pp. 158.
17. Lader D, Hopkins G. Contraception and sexual health 2007/08. Dyffryn: Office for National Statistics; 2007.
18. De Bastos M, Stegeman BH, Rosendaal FR, Van Hylckama Vlieg A, Helmerhorst FM, Stijnen T, et al. Combined oral contraceptives: venous thrombosis. Cochrane Database Syst Rev. 2014;3:CD010813.
19. Jang MJ, Bang SM, Oh D. Incidence of venous thromboembolism in Korea: from the Health Insurance Review and Assessment Service database. J Thromb Haemost. 2011;9:85-91.

20. Wu CQ, Grandi SM, Filion KB, Abenhaim HA, Joseph L, Eisenberg MJ. Drospirenone-containing oral contraceptive pills and the risk of venous and arterial thrombosis: a systematic review. BJOG. 2013;120(7):801-10.
21. Larivee N, Suissa S, Khosrow-Khavar T, Fillion KB. Drospirenone-containing oral contraceptive pills and the risk of venous and arterial thrombosis: a systematic review. BJOG. 2017;124(10):1490-9.
22. Dinger J, Bardenheuer K, Heinemann K. Cardiovascular and general safety of a 24-day regimen of drospirenone-containing combined oral contraceptives: final results from the international active surveillance study of women taking oral contraceptives. Contraception. 2014;89:253-63.
23. Committee on Gynecologic Practice. ACOG Committee Opinion Number 540: risk of venous thromboembolism among users of drospirenone-containing oral contraceptive pills depending on age lies between 2 and 20 per million. Obstet Gynecol. 2012;120(5):1239-42.
24. Arowojolu AO, Gallo MF, Lopez LM, Grimes DA. Combined oral contraceptive pills for treatment of acne. Cochrane Database Syst Rev. 2012;6:CD004425.
25. Clinical guidelines. Committee Opinion: Risk of venous thrombosis among users of Drospirenone containing. OCP. 2012;540:2-9.
26. Baldwin MK, Jensen JT. Contraception during the perimenopause. Maturitas. 2013;76:235-42.
27. Hong JS, Kang HC, Lee SH, Kim J. Long-term trend in the incidence of acute myocardial infarction in Korea: 1997-2007. Korean Circ J. 2009;39:467-76.
28. Marchbanks PA, McDonald JA, Wilson HG, Folger SG, Mandel MG, Daling JR, et al. Oral contraceptives and the risk of breast cancer. N Engl J Med. 2002;346:2025-32.
29. Gierisch JM, Coeytaux RR, Urrutia RP, Havrilesky LJ, Moorman PG, Lowery WJ, et al. Oral contraceptive use and risk of breast, cervical, colorectal, and endometrial cancers: a systematic review. Cancer Epidemiol Biomarkers Prev. 2013;22:1931-43.
30. Beaber E, Buist DS, Barlow WE, Malone KE, Reed SD, Li CL. Recent oral contraceptive use by formulation and breast cancer risk among women 20 to 49 years of age. Cancer Res. 2014;74:4078-89.
31. Hannaford PC, Selvaraj S, Elliot AM, Angus V, Iversen L, Lee AJ. Cancer risk among users of oral contraceptive: cohort data from the Royal College of General Practitioner's oral contraceptive study. BMJ. 2007;335:651.
32. Collaborative Group on Epidemiological Studies on Endometrial Cancer. Endometrial cancer and oral contraceptives: an individual participant meta-analysis of 27,276 women with endometrial cancer from 36 epidemiological studies. Lancet Oncol. 2015;16:1061-70.
33. Mantha S, Karp R, Raghavan V, Terrin N, Bauer KA, Zwicker JI. Assessing the risk of venous thromboembolic events in women taking progestin-only contraception: a meta-analysis. BMJ. 2012;345:e4944.
34. Newton J, Tacchi D. Long-term use of copper intrauterine devices. A statement from the Medical Advisory Committee of the Family Planning Association and the National Association of Family Planning Doctors. Lancet. 1990;335:1322-3.
35. Faculty of Sexual and Reproductive Healthcare Clinical Effectiveness Unit. FSRH clinical guidance: contraception for women over 40. London: FSRH; 2010.
36. Cancer Research UK. Uterine cancer (C54–C55), average number of new cases per year and age-specific incidence rates per 100,000 population, females, UK 2012–2014. London: Cancer Research UK; 2016.
37. Nappi RE, Merki-Feld GS, Terreno E, Pellegrinelli A, Viana MJ. Hormonal contraception in women with migraine: is progestogen-only contraception a better choice? J Headache Pain. 2013;14:66.
38. Farley TM, Rosenberg MJ, Rowe PJ, Chen JH, Meirik O. Intrauterine devices and pelvic inflammatory disease: an international perspective. Lancet. 1992;339:785-8.

39. Lee NC, Rubin GL, Borucki R. The intrauterine device and pelvic inflammatory disease revisited: new results from the Women's Health Study. Obstet Gynecol. 1988;72:1-6.
40. Piaggio G, Kapp N, von Hertzen H. Effect on pregnancy rates of the delay in the administration of levonorgestrel for emergency contraception: a combined analysis of four WHO trials. Contraception. 2011;84(1):35-9.
41. Faculty of Sexual and Reproductive Healthcare. Intrauterine contraception: Clinical effectiveness unit. London: Faculty of Sexual and Reproductive Healthcare; 2015.
42. Huang Y, Jensen JT, Brache V, Cochon L, Williams A, Miranda MJ, et al. A randomized study on pharmacodynamic effects of vaginal rings delivering the progesterone receptor modulator ulipristal acetate: research for a novel estrogen-free, method of contraception. Contraception. 2014;90:565-74.
43. OCON Medical Ltd. Safe and hormone free birth control: IUBTM copper pearls. [online] Available from: http://www.oconmed.com/en/support/brochures [Last accessed March, 2021].
44. Davis A, Godwin A, Lippman J, Olson W, Kafrissen M. Triphasic norgestimate-ethinyl estradiol for treating dysfunctional uterine bleeding. Obstet Gynecol. 2000;96(6):913-20.
45. Fraser IS, Jensen J, Schaefers M, Mellinger U, Parke S, Serrani M. Normalization of blood loss in women with heavy menstrual bleeding treated with an oral contraceptive containing estradiol valerate/dienogest. Contraception. 2012;86(2):96-101.
46. Kwiecien M, Edelman A, Nichols MD, Jensen JT. Bleeding patterns and patient acceptability of standard or continuous dosing regimens of a low-dose oral contraceptive: a randomized trial. Contraception. 2003;67:9-13.
47. Shargil AA. Hormone replacement therapy in perimenopausal women with a triphasic contraceptive compound: a three-year prospective study. Int J Fertil. 1985;30:15, 18-28.
48. Kritz-Silverstein D, Barrett-Connor E. Bone mineral density in postmenopausal women as determined by prior oral contraceptive use. Am J Public Health. 1993;83:100-2.
49. Shifren JL, Gass ML, NAMS Recommendations for Clinical Care of Midlife Women Working Group. The North American Menopause Society recommendations for clinical care of midlife women. Menopause. 2014;21:1038-62.
50. American College of Obstetrics and Gynecologists. Management of Anovulatory Bleeding (ACOG Practice Bulletin 14). Washington, DC: American College of Obstetricians and Gynecologists; 2000.

Skin Care and Menopause

CHAPTER

■ INTRODUCTION

Menopause is defined as a permanent irreversible cessation of menses brought by decline in ovarian follicular activity. Hormonal alteration results in various physical, psychological, and sexual changes in menopausal women. When menopause sets in as a turning point in life, there will be decline in skin qualities.

■ PATHOPHYSIOLOGY OF SKIN CHANGES DURING MENOPAUSE

The Importance of Hormones on the Skin

Ovarian failure and the resulting hormonal changes during menopause affect almost all aspects of women's health and may present with signs and symptoms in nearly every system in the body. Symptoms are experienced differently according to ethnic, educational, and sociocultural variability.

Estrogens are essential for skin hydration because they increase production of glycosaminoglycans, promote an increased production of sebum, increase water retention, improve barrier function of the stratum corneum, and optimize the surface area of corneocytes. As a result, concerns about dry skin are more frequent among menopausal women who are not taking hormone replacement therapy (HRT).[3] Decreased estrogen reduces the polymerization of glycosaminoglycans, while elastin experiences granular degeneration and fragmentation, forming cystic spaces. In addition, there is a reduction in the microvasculature and thinning of the epidermis.[1,2]

Albright et al.[17] noted that the skin of menopausal women with osteoporosis showed considerable atrophy, a finding subsequently supported by a study from Brincat et al.[18] In menopausal women, the decrease in estrogen promotes a reduction in type I and type III collagen and a reduction in the type III collagen to type I collagen ratio compared with nonmenopausal women.[4] Healthy skin is made up of type I collagen (80%, responsible for strength) to type III collagen (15%, responsible for elasticity).[3] However, a decrease in androgens is partially responsible for the reduction in sebum secretion, xerosis, and skin thinning or atrophy, accompanied by a reduction in blood vessels, oxygenation, and nutrition of the skin, as well as increased transepidermal water loss.[5,6] Regarding skin annexes, the decrease in estrogen causes a reduction in axillary and pubic hair. The reduction in elastic fibers results in a loss of firmness and elasticity. Moreover, with a relative predominance of androgenic hormones, vellus hair may be replaced by thicker hair.[7]

Anagen hair have estrogen receptors in both sexes. In contrast to the α-receptor, the β-receptor largely is expressed in the papillary dermis and the hair's bulb region; this expression could account for the occurrence of androgenetic alopecia in menopausal women. These receptors are not expressed in telogen hair, and their role in regulating the hair cycle is unknown. The aging of the follicular unit, resulting from the reduction of active melanocytes, promotes the appearance of gray hair. It is estimated that in 50% of men and women, half of their hair will be gray by 50 years of age. The age of onset for graying hair appears to be influenced by heredity and ethnicity. Unlike the skin, hair aging is more affected by intrinsic than extrinsic factors.

In women, hormonal changes during menopause are the main source of alterations in hair characteristics. The identification of high concentrations of hydrogen peroxide and low levels of catalase in the stems of gray hair has shed light on the biochemistry of hair whitening and opened new possibilities for its prevention and treatment. A change in the balance of oxidation/reduction reactions may lead to DNA damage and melanocyte apoptosis.

The Influence of HRT on Skin Changes in Postmenopausal Women

The importance of estrogens in maintenance of skin health offers the possibility that HRT could reduce the menopausal signs of atrophy (thinning), dry skin, and wrinkles. Moreover, one observational study in >3,000 women found that compared to nonusers, HRT use was associated with a statistically significant reduction in dry skin and wrinkling but not atrophy.[15]

Hormone replacement therapy appears to boast dermal collagen levels and thereby improves skin health. This has been the subject of several trials,[14] in which all but one demonstrated an improvement in collagen levels. It has been suggested that HRT was ineffective in one trial because the women had been amenorrheic for a short period of time (between 4 months and 2 years) and that any hypoestrogenic effects would have been small during this initial period of time.[15] The longest study of topical HRT continued for 4.8 years and used 0.06% estradiol gel or transdermal patches to maintain a daily estradiol dose of 1.5 mg. The trial observed increase of skin thickness between 7 and 15% in several areas of the body.[16] In contrast, a randomized, double-blind trial with oral conjugated estrogen therapy detected a 30% increase in dermal thickness after only 12 months.[17]

An increase in skin hydration has been demonstrated after 6 months use of topical 0.01% estradiol and 0.3% estriol for 6 months.[18] Although the mechanism through which estrogens increase skin hydration is unclear, studies in mice indicate that estradiol increases the level of hyaluronic acid and thereby the water content of the skin.[19]

Reducing wrinkles—collagen is broken down in the skin by a group of enzymes termed metalloproteinases, which have an important role in tissue repair and remodeling. A reduction in the amount and integrity of collagen within the dermis leads to progressive slackness of the skin, a loss of elasticity, and subsequent wrinkle formation. This process is exacerbated on sun-exposed areas of skin such as the face, which is subject to photo-aging.

HRT can improve or not the appearance of wrinkles on sunexposed areas of the body is equivocal. One study found that HRT was able to reduce skin slackness (and potentially wrinkle appearance, but this was not assessed). Another study using Premarin cream (0.625 mg conjugated estrogens) in women aged between 52 and 70 for 24 weeks did produce a significant improvement in fine wrinkles. A third study in women using HRT for at least 5 years also produced improvements in skin elasticity with less pronounced wrinkling. In contrast, however, other trials have failed to demonstrate any benefits. In the largest of these studies, Phillips et al. enrolled 485 patients using oral HRT for 48 weeks and found no difference in facial wrinkling. Similarly, Yoon et al., using topical estrone 1% or placebo on sun-exposed skin for 24 weeks, found no difference compared to placebo. In a third study, application of topical estradiol 0.05% cream to photo-exposed skin (face) for 30 days did not observe changes in the expression of metalloproteinase-1 enzyme (which degrades collagen).

More recent studies have demonstrated that alternatives to HRT, such as selective estrogen receptor modulators (SERMs) (e.g., raloxifene), are able to increase collagen synthesis in dermal fibroblasts and increase skin elasticity.

■ PHYSIOLOGICAL CHANGES OF MENOPAUSE

- *Age spots and signs of sun-damaged skin*: Age spots and larger areas of darker skin can appear on face, hands, neck, arms, or chest, if there is an excessive sun exposure without sun protection. Skin cancer and precancerous skin growths also become more common.
- *Bruise easily*: As estrogen levels fall, skin becomes thinner. Thin skin bruises more easily.
- *Dry skin*: In menopause, skin loses some ability to hold water, so skin can get quite dry. This can be especially noticeable when the air is dry.
- *Facial hair*: As levels of female hormones fall, you can see unwanted hair under your chin and along your jawline or above your lip. Hair loss on your head.
- *Thinning of hair*: At menopause, many women notice thinning hair on their head. The first sign may be a widening part. Some women find that their hairline starts to recede.
- *Jowls, slack skin, and wrinkles*: In menopause, skin quickly loses collagen. Studies show that women's skin loses about 30% of its collagen during the first 5 years of menopause. After that, the decline is more

gradual. Women lose about 2% of their collagen ever year for the next 20 years.

As collagen diminishes, our skin loses its firmness and begins to sag. Jowls appear. Permanent lines run from the tip of the nose to the corners of the mouth. Wrinkles that used to appear only with a smile or frown become visible all the time. Later, the tip of the nose dips, pouches under eyes. Large pores also are due to lack of skin firmness.

- *Pimples and other types of acne*: As levels of female hormones drop before and during menopause, some women develop teenage-like acne.
- *Wounds heal more slowly*: Hormones play an important role in healing our skin. When hormone levels fall, skin takes longer time to heal.

■ MANAGEMENT OF PHYSIOLOGICAL CHANGES OF MENOPAUSE

- *Antiaging cream or broad-spectrum sunscreen*: Apply sunscreen every day before going outdoors. To give your skin the protection it needs, use a broad-spectrum sunscreen with SPF 30 or higher. Apply it to all skin that clothing would not cover.

  This can help fade age spots, prevent new spots from forming, and reduce your risk of getting skin cancer. Apply a broad-spectrum sunscreen with SPF 30 or higher every day. While this cannot thicken your skin, it can prevent further thinning. You should apply sunscreen to your face, hands, neck, and any other area that clothing would not cover. And you should do this every day, even in winter.

- *The following can help combat dry skin*:
  - Wash with a mild cleanser instead of soap. For mature skin, soap can be too drying. Skip the deodorant bars.
  - Apply moisturizer after bathing and throughout the day when your skin feels dry. A moisturizer with hyaluronic acid or glycerin can be especially helpful.
  - *Ceramides and retinoids cream*: Women need to repair their epidermis by moisturizers that contain ceramides, as well as a broad-spectrum sunscreen, and retinoids are used to slow down photoaging and repair the epidermis by stimulating new collagen growth.

- *Battling acne*: During menopause, women begin breaking out with acne on the lower section. of the face, depending upon the severity of a woman's acne, oral antibiotics, hormonal therapy, and low-dose oral contraceptive pills that often help with adult hormonal acne, as well as spironolactone, which is another prescription medication, are advised. And there are many topical medications, for example, metronidazole, as well as medications that contain azelaic acid.

- *Unwanted hair*: There are many ways to remove excessive facial hair. Depilatory creams, plucking, waxing or shaving are some of the ways, and there is laser hair reduction, which is extremely effective.

- *Alopecia*: Treatment for hair loss depends on the cause. If your hair loss is due to menopause, your dermatologist may recommend minoxidil, laser treatment, or both.[14]

If you have already lost a considerable amount of hair, a hair transplant may be an option.

PRIMARY SKIN DISORDERS OF MENOPAUSE AND MANAGEMENT

Pruritus

Pruritus is the primary skin concern in women older than 65 years. Given that xerosis is the most prominent cause of pruritus, consider the possible role of menopause-related transepidermal water loss.[5]

Types of Itching during Menopause

Xerosis: Skin becomes drier and less elastic during menopause, people may be more sensitive to products, such as soaps and detergents. Others experience a rare type of paraesthesia known as formication during menopause. Formication is having the sensation of insects crawling under the skin.

Genital itching: Reduced levels of estrogen mean that vaginal problems may arise or get worse during or after menopause. People may notice vaginal itching more often during menopause. Vaginal itching is called vulvar pruritus.

The following factors can also cause vaginal itching:
- Irritation from soaps or detergents
- Inflammation
- Vaginal, vulvar, or rarely, cervical cancers.

Regardless of the underlying cause, however, some general measures are recommended for managing pruritus in menopausal women such as using low-pH moisturizers daily, preferably after bathing; keeping nails short; wearing loose and light clothing; maintaining a comfortable ambient temperature; using humidifiers or air-conditioning devices; restricting bathing time; and avoiding hot water and high-pH sanitizers.[8]

Hyperhidrosis

Night sweats, hyperhidrosis, and hot flashes (flushing) are common concerns in 35-50% of perimenopausal women and in 30-80% of postmenopausal women. Menopausal hyperhidrosis is classified as secondary hyperhidrosis, the symptoms of which may be alleviated by HRT, suggesting that the cause is decreasing levels of estrogen.[9]

In addition to HRT, other treatments such as gabapentin, serotonin-norepinephrine reuptake inhibitors, and acupuncture are used to treat menopausal hyperhidrosis.

Senile Alopecia

Starting at 50 years of age, scalp hair show varying degrees of change in pigmentation, growth, and diameter. Despite the normal ratio of telogen to anagen hair, there may be a considerable reduction in follicular density. The clinical distinction between senile alopecia and androgenetic alopecia can be challenging, and the conditions may coexist.[10] 2–5% minoxidil solution,[11] which is able to interrupt hair loss or induce mild-to-moderate regrowth in 60% of patients with female pattern hair loss (FPHL).

Androgenetic Alopecia

Up to 50% of women experience androgenetic alopecia, or FPHL, during their lives.[16] It is the main cause of hair loss in women, and women in perimenopause are the most affected. Hair regrowth is difficult when treatment is not instituted early in perimenopausal FPHL. The pathogenesis involves a progressive reduction in the hair cycle, resulting in shrinkage of the hair follicles. Unlike the pathogenesis of androgenetic alopecia in men, little is known about the role of androgens in FPHL. The measurement of androgen levels is not recommended in the absence of symptoms of virilization or in the absence of abnormal clinical patterns or progression.

Female pattern hair loss primarily is treated with a 2–5% minoxidil solution, which is able to interrupt hair loss or induce mild-to-moderate regrowth in 60% of patients with FPHL. The effectiveness of the treatment should only be assessed after 1 year of use. Contact dermatitis is the main adverse effect, but its incidence may be reduced by up to 82% by using vehicles that do not contain propylene glycol. If the use of minoxidil solution is not possible, good results also have been reported with antiandrogen medications, such as spironolactone. These drugs are especially useful in cases of hyperandrogenism.

Conventional doses of finasteride 1 mg daily, as used in men, have shown discrepant results in menopausal women. Improvement of FPHL has been shown in studies using doses of 2.5 mg or higher for a minimum of 12 months. The use of dutasteride, an inhibitor of 5α-reductases I and II, promotes greater inhibition (100%) of dihydrotestosterone activity than finasteride (70%) in men; however, it has not yet been approved by the US Food and Drug Administration for treatment in women.

Impaired Wound Healing

Wound healing also is affected by aging. Delays in healing may be more closely related to the decrease in estrogen levels than to intrinsic aging. A comparison between the expression of genes associated with healing in young and elderly men showed that most of the genes are regulated exclusively by estrogen, which could explain the higher incidence of chronic ulcers in elderly men compared to women. However, menopausal women also are at risk for development of chronic ulcers. Ashcroft et al. showed that the use of topical estrogen accelerates the healing of acute[19] incisional wounds by increasing transforming growth factor β.

Healing of the oral mucosa is associated with a higher rate of complications and longer recovery time in women than in men. Estrogens produce anti-inflammatory effects, whereas progesterone demonstrates a proinflammatory effect. Testosterone has anti-inflammatory effects and is able to modify the proinflammatory state in the oral mucosae of menopausal women. Wound healing in menopausal women who are not receiving HRT tends to be slower than in those who are receiving HRT. Age is not necessarily an important factor in wound healing. Premenopausal and younger women have shown no notable differences in healing. Nevertheless, after menopause, differences in wound healing have been found, indicating that hormonal status may be more crucial to wound healing than age.

Atrophic Vulvovaginitis[12,13]

Thinning (atrophy) of vaginal skin including the entrance to the vagina (vestibule). The vulva is less affected (it has fewer estrogen receptors than the vagina) symptoms include itchiness, tenderness, a burning sensation, painful intercourse (dyspareunia), and painful urination.

Vulvovaginal Candidias

Vulvar Lichen Sclerosis

A chronic skin disease that mainly affects the anogenital area.

Signs and symptoms include:
- Itching and irritation
- White, thinned, wrinkled skin
- Recurrent fissures of posterior fourchette (vaginal tears)
- Painful intercourse (dyspareunia)
- Labial fusion.

Menopausal Flushing

It occurs in 70–85% of women throughout the perimenopausal stage.

Keratoderma Climacteric

It is the thickening of skin on the palms and soles.

Common Dermatoses with No Hormonal Associations

Brittle Nail Syndrome

Brittle nail syndrome (BNS) affects 20% of the population with a female-to-male ratio of 2:1. The pathogenesis of BNS involves factors that affect the adhesion of corneocytes to the nail plate and alter nail formation from its matrix; the former process produces onychoschizia, whereas the latter leads to onychorrhexis.

Management of BNS requires the correction of the precipitating cause by hydration of the nail blade, cuticle, and proximal nail folds, preferably under occlusion. Supplementation with biotin is considered highly effective by many researchers. In a retrospective study, the use of biotin for 6 months improved BNS in 63% (22/35) of patients. Recommended doses generally are >2.5 mg daily. The use of 10% urea in nail polish once or twice daily showed that both regimens improved the morphology, consistency, and reflectiveness of the nail plate.

Frontal Fibrosing Alopecia

Frontal fibrosing alopecia has a tendency to affect menopausal women. Frontal fibrosing alopecia is a slow, progressive, and lymphocytic cicatricial alopecia that produces symmetrical frontal or temporal recession but rarely affects other areas of the scalp. It often is associated with nonscarring alopecia of body hair or eyebrows. The cicatricial area is atrophic, pale, and surrounded by hyperpigmented skin due to long-term sun damage.

Many investigators believe it is a variant of lichen planopilaris. Others suggest the possibility that hormonal changes characteristic of perimenopause contribute to triggering the disease. Some cases show a partial response to finasteride or dutasteride. Furthermore, the lymphocytic inflammatory component of the disorder has been treated with immunomodulators, topical and intralesional corticosteroids, and hydroxychloroquine.

Telogen Effluvium

Telogen effluvium (TE) is the premature transformation of hair from the anagen phase to the telogen phase. Considered a symptom of an underlying condition (e.g., endocrine, nutritional, and autoimmune disorders) rather than a full diagnosis in itself, TE is characterized by diffuse hair loss confirmed by a pull test in which >5 hair are removed from the scalp on tugging a section of 25-50 hair. If there is concurrent TE in women with androgenetic alopecia, more severe hair loss has been reported. There may be concerns of dysesthesia of the scalp (trichodynia), especially in patients with emotional stress.

Most often diagnosed in women, TE in its acute form is even more common in menopausal women and lasts <6 months. The acute form of TE is secondary to hemorrhage, high fever, surgery, drug use, systemic diseases, diet, or great psychological stress and typically occurs 1-3 months after the primary event. The most common cause of iron deficiency at menopausal transition is malabsorption or chronic gastrointestinal bleeding. Ferritin levels below 40 µg/L are associated with hair loss with a 98% specificity and sensitivity. Low serum levels of vitamin B_{12} or vitamin D also are considered important factors.

Chronic TE (i.e., lasting >6 months) predominantly occurs in women aged 40-60 years, and its onset is abrupt. Chronic TE is considered a diagnosis of exclusion. In 30% of cases of chronic diffuse hair loss lasting longer than 6 months, the cause is unknown. The pathogenesis is poorly understood, though it is assumed to result from a reduced duration of the anagen growth phase in the absence of shrinking hair follicles.

Patient education is the most important aspect of TE management. The aim of treatment is to reduce hair loss and correct the precipitating factors. Even if the underlying cause is corrected, hair loss may continue for up to 6 months with the desired cosmetic regrowth occurring after only 12-18 months. In acute secondary TE, the course of the disease is self-limited, and correction of the causal factor is sufficient. In chronic diffuse loss, identification of causal factors is more difficult, and treatment involves adequate nutrition (i.e., at least 1,200 calories daily including 9.8 mg/kg body weight of protein) and multivitamin supplementation, minoxidil, and even antiandrogen medications.

Trichotillomania

Trichotillomania is the compulsive behavior of plucking strands of hair and is considered to be a poor adaptive response to stress. Although trichotillomania most commonly occurs in children, adolescents, and young adults, in older adults it is more often associated with psychopathology and is markedly more common in women. The condition usually is refractory to treatment, and although the scalp usually is the primary focus of the behavior, eventually patients may pluck body hair. Menopausal women also may present with trichoteiromania in which hair loss is secondary to repeated friction that has fractured the hair shaft; this condition often is associated with scalp dysesthesia. Trichotillomania is considered an obsessive-compulsive disorder, whereas trichoteiromania needs further investigation because it can occur secondary to many psychiatric disorders. The specific psychotherapeutic and pharmacologic treatments likely will depend on the underlying cause of the disease.

WHAT TREATMENT IS AVAILABLE FOR MENOPAUSAL SYMPTOMS?

Treatment of Skin Disorders in Menopausal Women

- *Classic HRT:* Several studies have used histologic analysis or ultrasonography to show that estrogens used in HRT thicken the skin or increase collagen content, whether given orally, topically, or transdermally. In a randomized, double-blind study comparing topical estrogen versus glycolic acid, 6 months of estrogen use on only one side of the face promoted a 23% increase in epidermal thickness ($P = 0.00458$), and the use of glycolic acid stimulated a 27% increase ($P = 0.00467$). The combined use of estrogen and glycolic acid prompted a 38% increase in epidermal thickness ($P = 0.000181$), with significant differences observed for all groups compared with the controls for the reversal of histologic markers of skin aging.

Finally, collagen synthesis also is increased as inferred by the increase in procollagen type I and II terminal peptides. HRT also affects the skin's ability to retain water and leads to a reduction in skin wrinkling; however, the effects of HRT on dyschromic alterations have not been well-studied. The numerous adverse effects of HRT, such as an increased incidence of cancer and cardiovascular morbidity, limit its use.

Hormone replacement therapy has been shown to prevent many of the signs and symptoms experienced in peri- and post-menopause, including urogenital and general skin and hair problems.

Estrogen cream is particularly useful for atrophic vulvovaginitis, and systemic absorption and side effects are minimal.

Other treatments for the genitourinary syndrome of menopause may include:
- Avoidance of soaps and harsh rubbing of the affected area to prevent further irritation of the skin
- Topical or oral antibiotics, if an infection is present
- Emollients and bland lubricants to keep the area moist
- Tricyclic antidepressants, such as amitriptyline, for neuropathic pain.

Considering all the evidence and taking into account that the safe limit for sun exposure that allows maximum synthesis of vitamin D without an increased risk for skin cancer remains unknown, the American Academy of Dermatology states that intentional exposure to the sun should not be considered a main source of sun exposure and the use of sunscreen should not be discouraged. Instead, the Academy recommends using dietary sources of vitamin D or artificial vitamin D supplementation at doses that vary by age—between 1 and 70 years, a dose of 600 IU daily is recommended; on average, women aged >50 years older are recommended a dose of 800 IU daily.

■ KEY MESSAGES

- Hormonal alteration results in various physical, psychological, and sexual changes in menopausal women. Skin disorders are quite common during menopause but often overlooked. For early and effective preventive therapeutic approach, knowledge about physiology is important.
- Estrogens are essential for skin hydration because they increase production of glycosaminoglycans, promote an increased production of sebum, increase water retention, improve barrier function of the stratum corneum, and optimize the surface area of corneocytes.

- Physiological changes of menopause are age spots, bruise easily, dry skin, facial hair, thinning of hair, jowls, slack skin, and wrinkles, pimples and other types of acne, and slowly healing wounds.
- Management of physiological changes of menopause is mainly using anti-aging and sunscreen creams and using moisturizer to combat dry skin.
- Pruritus is the primary skin concern in women older than 65 years. General measures are recommended for managing pruritus in menopausal women such as using low-pH moisturizers daily, preferably after bathing; keeping nails short; wearing loose and light clothing.

    They should maintain a comfortable ambient temperature; using humidifiers or air-conditioning devices; restrict bathing time; and avoid hot water and high-pH sanitizers.
- Hormone replacement therapy has been shown to prevent many of the signs and symptoms experienced in peri- and post-menopause, including urogenital and general skin and hair problems. But evidence of direct effect of menopause hormone therapy on skin is still lacking.
- Though there are numerous treatment options for menopausal skin changes including pharmaceuticals, cosmetics treatments, lifestyle measures, topical retinoids, facial peel, botulinum neurotoxin, soft tissue fillers, and surgical procedures that can be employed to improve the appearance of the skin, treatment should be tailored to suit the women's individual need.

REFERENCES

1. Gilhar A, Ullmann Y, Karry R, Shalaginov R, Assy B, Serafimovich S, et al. Ageing of human epidermis: the role of apoptosis, Fas and telomerase. Br J Dermatol. 2004; 150(1):56-63.
2. Accorsi-Neto A, Haidar M, Simões R, Simões M, Soares J Jr, Baracat E. Effects of isoflavones on the skin of postmenopausal women: a pilot study. Clinics (Sao Paulo). 2009;64(6):505-10.
3. Shah MG, Maibach HI. Estrogen and skin. an overview. Am J Clin Dermatol. 2001;2(3):143-50.
4. Affinito P, Palomba S, Sorrentino C, Di Carlo C, Bifulco G, Arienzo MP, et al. Effects of postmenopausal hypoestrogenism on skin collagen. Maturitas. 1999;33(3):239-47.
5. Pérez-López FR. Androgens in menopausal women [in Spanish]. Med Clin (Barc). 2003;120:31-6.
6. Verdier-Sévrain S, Bonté F, Gilchrest B. Biology of estrogens in skin: implications for skin aging. Exp Dermatol. 2006;15(2):83-94.
7. Al-Azzawi F, Palacios S. Hormonal changes during menopause. Maturitas. 2009;63(2):135-7.
8. Patel T, Yosipovitch G. The management of chronic pruritus in the elderly. Skin Therapy Lett. 2010;15(8):5-9.
9. Paisley AN, Buckler HM. Investigating secondary hyperhidrosis. BMJ. 2010;341: c4475.
10. Chen W, Yang CC, Todorova A. Hair loss in elderly women. Eur J Dermatol. 2010; 20:145-51.

11. Rivera R, Guerra-Tapia A. Management of androgenetic alopecia in postmenopausal women [in Spanish]. Actas Dermosifiliogr. 2008;99(4):257-61.
12. Wines N, Willsteed E. Menopause and the skin. Australas J Dermatol. 2001;42: 149-60.
13. Kim HK, Kang SY, Chung YJ, Kim JH, Kim MR. The recent review of the genitourinary syndrome of menopause. J Menopausal Med. 2015;21(2):65-71.
14. White GM, Cox NH. Disorders of hair. In: White GM and Cox NH (Eds). Diseases of the Skin: A Color Atlas and Text, 2nd edition. China: Mosby Elsevier; 2006. pp. 588-9.
15. Dunn LB, Damesyn M, Moore AA, Reuben DB, Greendale GA. Does estrogen prevent skin aging? Results from the First National Health and Nutrition Examination Survey (NHANES I). Arch Dermatol. 1997;133(3):339-42.
16. Chen W, Yang CC, Todorova A, Al Khuzaei S, Chiu HC, Worret WI, et al. Hair loss in elderly women. Hair loss in elderly women. Eur J Dermatol. 2010;20(2):145-51.
17. Albright F, Smith PH, Richardson AM. Postmenopausal osteoporosis. its clinical features. JAMA. 1941;116:2465-74.
18. Brincat M, Kabalan S, Studd JW, Moniz CF, de Trafford J, Montgomery J. A study of the decrease of skin collagen content, skin thickness, and bone mass in the postmenopausal woman. Obstet Gynecol. 1987;70(6):840-5.
19. Ashcroft GS, Dodsworth J, van Boxtel E, Tarnuzzer RW, Horan MA, Schultz GS, et al. Estrogen accelerates cutaneous wound healing associated with an increase in TGF-beta1 levels. Nat Med. 1997;3(11):1209-15.

Mental Health and Menopause

CHAPTER

■ INTRODUCTION

The menopause can impact on a woman's health both physically and psychologically, primarily due to the depletion of the hormone estrogen in the body. Mental health through menopause transition can be debilitating to the women, her family and society. In addition to hot flushes, the sweats, tiredness and vaginal dryness, some women also experience emotional and psychological symptoms such as anxiety, sleeplessness, irritability, poor concentration and low self-esteem, which can often be mistaken for depression. Even they might present symptoms mimicking depression.

The National Institute for Health and Care Excellence (NICE, 2015) defines *menopause* as when a woman stops having periods as she reaches the end of her natural reproductive life. This is not usually abrupt but a gradual process during which women experience perimenopause changes before reaching postmenopause when periods become irregular and then stop with the end of fertility. A woman is postmenopausal when she has not had a period for 12 months.

There are many symptoms of the menopause including flushes, mood changes, "brain fog", vaginal symptoms, bloating and joint pains. Often women may not relate them to the menopause.

Emotions related to life course are different to clinical symptoms of depression but can easily be mistaken for each other.

Women experiencing similar symptoms such as low mood, anxiety and "brain fog" may be linked to hormonal changes in the body, and crucially, can be treated and will pass. Many women of menopausal age are affected by mental health issues. But whereas women are prepared for hot flushes and sweats they are not necessarily expecting symptoms such as low mood or anxiety, which can have a huge impact on home and work life. Therefore we need to provide special attention to this group of women.

■ EFFECT OF HORMONE DEFICIENCY

The hormonal changes of perimenopause and menopause during the first few years after the menopause can cause emotions to change quite quickly. Estrogen has positive relation with neurotransmitter of the brain. But due to menopause, estrogen hormone deficiency has negative impact on mental health. Emotions can swing from joy one moment to anger and irritability the next in the blink of eye.

Identifying what is a menopausal symptom and what are "true" mood changes, depression or anxiety can be confusing. Often anxiety symptoms get worse with perimenopause. What might start as a hot flush might lead to an anxiety attack.

In turn, the symptoms of menopause, such as hot flushes and night sweats, can affect mood and make some women feel depressed. Many women kept awake at night because of night sweats find they are exhausted, cannot think clearly and feel more negative because they have had poor quality sleep.

Depression and depressed mood around the time of expected menopause 51-52 years is more likely to occur because of factors other than menopause, including:

- Prior episodes of depression
- Significant stress in life
- A negative attitude to things happening in life
- Dissatisfaction with your relationships
- Low self-esteem
- Poor body image
- Poor lifestyle such as little exercise or a high intake of alcohol.

Emotional health around the menopause is also more likely to be influenced by previous experiences of prior traumatic events, for example, past abuse. Women often seek counseling at menopause and might want to work through traumas they have previously experienced. This time of life seems to allow things to come to the surface.

■ WOMEN'S PSYCHOLOGY

Mental and emotional health is influenced by many factors. In general, women have been found to be twice as likely as men to experience an affective disorder and anxiety disorder.[1,2] Hormones and biological factors such as menopause in the increased incidence of mood disorders in women. Interestingly, however, researchers have found that the prevalence of depression decreases with age and was experienced more by women in the childbearing years,[3-5] for example, in a large Australian population study, women aged 18-24 years experienced the highest prevalence of depression at 11%, while 7% of women aged 45-54 years experienced depression.[3] It appears that women also believe that hormones account for their experiences of depression and anxiety. Many menopausal women present to their practitioner for the first time with low mood and anxiety symptoms in their mid to late forties believing that they are caused by menopause. However, after a thorough history is taken, it is often discovered that the woman has experienced these symptoms previously. Women may feel that they can finally report they are depressed and anxious because menopause has legitimized these symptoms.

■ DIAGNOSIS

Thorough history taking highlighting the predisposing factors, clinical examination and listening from the menopause women are most important. We need to know details about sleep pattern as inadequate sleep has tremendous effect on adverse mental health. Not much tests are required but for diagnosis we need to do several tests to exclude the differential diagnosis. Particularly if the woman comes with this complain and having premature menopause.

■ MANAGEMENT

Mid-life is a time of transition and stressful life events from divorce to a second career, combined with physical changes can result in feeling overwhelmed. A number of studies have identified that menopause significantly impacts mood and mental health, including higher stress levels and depression.

Anxiety and panic attacks are also reported during menopause. Clear diagnosis need to be made and management needs multiprofessional collaboration.

More emphasis should be given to the hormonal changes and physical symptoms such as sleeplessness, affecting biological functioning especially for women with bipolar illness. To get the maximum benefits women should be managed by the gynecologists (for hormone therapy), psychologist and the counselors. Due to menopause, women with schizophrenia and depression may be at increased risk of an episode as their production of estrogen decreases. Some antipsychotic medications such as Sulpiride and Risperidone may cause periods to stop, which can be misdiagnosed as menopause. Therefore they need special care from our psychiatrist colleagues.

It would appear that at the same time women experience changes in their body associated with physiological aspects of menopause as it is also important to account for the psychological and social influences on their lives. Endocrine status cannot be used to predict whether women will experience negative psychological functioning; rather psychological morbidity is influenced by many factors and requires a multifaceted approach to its treatment.

Taking time to establish a therapeutic relationship with the woman who is menopausal may help to make her treatment and the experience of menopause more positive. It is important to assess thoughts and feelings about personal psychological vulnerability and her mental attitude. We need to ask women about the roles they have in their life if they are satisfied with these roles even we need to encourage them to seek new roles and try something they have always wanted to do—this could be enrolling in an adult education course, performing volunteer work, social engagement, etc. Also we should assess the social background of the menopausal patient, about the culture a woman comes from and how it might influence her experience of menopause.[6]

Improvement of interpersonal relationships, role in the family, and engaging in the society are the part of treatment. Many menopausal women have reported that they want further education and information, support, validation and for someone to take the time to listen to their individual experience.[7]

Some women will need further counseling, and referral to a qualified psychologist in combination with the treatment provided by a physician should be considered as an option.

Managing Anxiety, Depression and Sleep

Anxiety, depression and sleep are interlinked as anxiety and depression can trigger sleep problems and sleeplessness can make anxiety and depression worse.

Lack of sleep can affect mental well-being, cognitive function and cardiac health [NICE guideline (NG23) 2015 on Menopause].

Sleep disturbances are common throughout the perimenopause, menopause and postmenopause. These can include: Difficulty in getting to sleep; difficulty in staying asleep; poor quality sleep; waking early; and fatigue during the day. Night sweats can make sleep uncomfortable and can cause regular waking.

Sleep disturbances can be caused by lack of estrogen, causing hot flushes and sweats. Mood can also be affected and anxiety can lead to difficulty getting to sleep and early morning wakening. Other consequences of estrogen decline such as bladder problems, joint aches and pains can also cause sleep disturbance. Progesterone decline at menopause may also contribute to sleep disturbances, as it can be sleep inducing and can have calming relaxing effects—the lack of this can contribute to anxiety and restless agitation. Melatonin is another important hormone for sleep and this decreases with ages, it is also influenced by estrogen and progesterone levels.

Treatments for poor sleep include: Adequate exercise (not before bed), healthy diet and managing stress. Maintaining a regular bedtime and trying not to nap in the day can also help. Cognitive behavioral therapy can reduce menopausal symptoms such as low mood, anxiety and sleep disturbance. Menopause hormone therapy (MHT) can improve sleep particularly for women who are having hot flushes and sweats, and those women who are suffering from insomnia.

Menopause is not a high risk for mental health issues; it is a time of psychological stress. For example, depression is more common in women than men resulting from hormonal changes such as:
- Premenstrual syndrome (PMS) or premenstrual dysphoric disorder (PMDD)
- Postnatal depression.

Around the menopause: It seems to be worse in the few years before periods stop. Women who have a history of reproductive depression are more susceptible around the menopause and it is important to note that estrogens are good for treating these women. Sadness, low mood and mood swings can also occur during the menopause but are distinct from depression, which is a diagnosable condition. It is normal to feel emotional about physical changes such as getting older, the impact of poor sleep and the loss of fertility, role changes such as children leaving home, looking after aging parents or other relatives, or facing the loss of parents. Menopause can signal a time to take stock of life and focus on the next stage. Emotions related to life course are different from clinical symptoms of depression, which may include:

- Low mood lasting 2 weeks or more
- Feeling hopeless or flat feeling tired
- Changes in appetite (comfort eating or loos of appetite)
- Worthlessness
- Changed or trouble in sleep patterns, feeling of dread, unease or agitation
- Trouble in concentrating or making decisions.

Women should be encouraged to seek help and if a woman has thoughts of harming herself seek help straight away.

Sleep disturbance: A distressing feature of hot flashes is that they are more common at night than during the day and are associated with arousal from sleep. However, women experience sleep disturbances even in the absence of hot flashes. The estimated prevalence of difficulty in sleeping based upon two longitudinal cohort studies was 32–40% in the early menopausal transition, increasing to 38–46% in the late transition.[8]

Anxiety and depression symptoms may also contribute to sleep disturbances; in one study, they were predictive of sleep disturbances.[9] In addition, perimenopausal women with hot flashes are more likely to be depressed.[10,11] Primary sleep disorders are also common in this population. They are more prone to suffer from sleep disturbances, sleep apnea, and restless legs syndrome (RLS).[9]

Thus, in peri- or postmenopausal women who report sleep disturbances, treating the vasomotor symptoms may decrease sleep disturbances, but this may not resolve all sleep problems, as there are many other things that can disturb sleep, such as primary sleep disorders, anxiety, and depression so those factors must be treated too.[9]

Insomnia is especially common in older adults and women. One-third to two-thirds of adults endorse insomnia symptoms of any severity and approximately 10–15% endorse chronic insomnia with daytime consequences.

Insomnia has a complex relationship with other medical and psychiatric disorders and is no longer considered "primary" or "secondary" depending on the presence or absence of an associated condition. Successful treatment requires attention to the insomnia itself as well as relevant comorbidities.

Approximately half of patients with chronic insomnia have a psychiatric disorder, and the majority of those with a psychiatric disorder have insomnia. Frequent comorbidities include mood disorders, substance use disorders, and post-traumatic stress disorder.

High-risk medical conditions for chronic insomnia include pulmonary disease, hypertension, diabetes, cancer, chronic pain, and heart failure.

Neurodegenerative disorders including dementia and Parkinson disease are frequently accompanied by sleep disturbances and chronic insomnia.

Medications and substances contribute to chronic insomnia in many patients. Commonly implicated classes include central nervous system stimulants, certain antidepressants, glucocorticoids, alcohol, tobacco, and caffeine. Insomnia symptoms commonly co-occur with other sleep disorders, especially sleep apnea, RLS, and circadian sleep-wake rhythm disorders.

Sequelae of insomnia include decreased quality-of-life, complaints of impaired daytime performance, and increased risk of medical and psychiatric comorbidities.

Generally we need to advice the women to go to bed and get up at the same time each day, sleep in dark quiet place at a comfortable temperature.

They should avoid large meal, caffeine, tea after evening, nicotine and smoking and they should practice exercise everyday not just before sleep.

They should maintain dim light bedroom with comfortable bed with no electronics or gadgets around.

They may practice mind body therapies, yoga and tai chi if they wish.

In resistant cases we may prescribe short-term melatonin agonists, benzodiazepines before referring to the psychiatrists.

■ ADVERSE OUTCOMES

Chronic insomnia has an adverse impact on daytime function and quality-of-life, and insomnia with objective short sleep duration is associated with increased cardiovascular risk and mortality.

Quality-of-life: Patients with insomnia report increased fatigue, sleepiness, confusion, tension, anxiety, and depression compared with controls.[12]

Cognitive function and performance: Patients with insomnia are almost universally concerned that their poor sleep has negative consequences on their performance of daily tasks and consistently report subjective performance deficits.[13,14]

Self-medication: Patients who do not receive treatment for insomnia frequently seek over-the-counter remedies and have an increased risk of substance abuse.[15]

Association with suicide: Insomnia symptoms have been associated with an increased risk for suicidal thoughts and behaviors. Some studies have suggested that the association is primarily mediated by underlying depression, while in other studies; the association is present even after adjusting for psychiatric comorbidities.[16]

Cardiovascular risk and mortality: Insomnia is associated with sympathetic nervous system activation, and a number of studies have shown an association between insomnia and elevated cardiovascular risk, including hypertension and myocardial infarction.[17-20] Menopause women are more prone to have sleeplessness, this chronic insomnia is associated with more cardiovascular disease.[21-23]

The physiological activation associated with chronic objective insomnia likely accounts for the association between insomnia and hypertension, cardiovascular disease, diabetes, and metabolic disorder.[24,25]

■ DEPRESSION

Symptoms of depressive disorders as defined by the DSM-IV (Diagnostic and Statistics Manual)—for example, changes to weight, fatigue and lethargy, increased negative thoughts, thoughts of suicide. Depression may be diagnosed in levels such as mild (low mood that comes and goes) to moderate (persistent low mood with some physical symptoms) to severe and clinical (persistent low mood with increased physical symptoms, increased thoughts of suicide and delusions) it is also helpful to ask women to keep a diary over a 3-month period to determine whether they are experiencing symptoms related to menstrual changes and the menopause or whether other factors such as family problems are more responsible for depressed mood due to the biopsychosocial nature of depression a multidimensional approach is necessary for effective treatment. Women presenting at the menopause with mild depression may benefit from hormone replacement therapy (MHT).[26-28] It would also be appropriate to consider psychological therapy with this patient, such as cognitive behavioral therapy (CBT). Moderate-to-severe and clinical depression has been found to benefit from antidepressants, in particular selective serotonin re-uptake inhibitors (SSRIs) along with psychological therapy and possibly MHT. It is important to note that if women are also taking MHT they may require a lower dose of antidepressant.[20] Treatment of depression should always integrate both biological and psychological modalities.

■ KEY MESSAGES

- Mental health through menopause transition can be debilitating to the women, her family and the society.
- The influence of endocrine function on the mood of the menopausal woman continues to be debated and researched.
- While many women present at the menopause with low mood, depression and anxiety, the reasons for these mood disorders cannot be attributed to menopause status alone.

- The influence of psychological factors, lifestyle, body image, interpersonal relationships, role, and sociocultural factors in predicting levels of depression and anxiety in the menopausal patient cannot be ignored.
- The role of psychosocial factors in the symptomatology of menopausal women and prematurely menopausal women are very important.
- The importance of understanding the individual menopausal experiences of women within the context of their lives while offering support, education, and validation need to be highlighted.
- The need for a multidimensional approach for treating the menopausal woman who presents with mood disorders must be ensured. As mental health left untreated or unattended, it can progress to more advanced noncommunicable disorder.
- It is important that women maintain a healthy diet and regular exercise after the menopause to minimize health problems and promote self-esteem and well-being.
- Symptoms (type and severity) and the age of menopause will guide the need for any treatment. However, holistic treatment involving multiprofessional team is the cornerstone of the treatment.
- Women must be informed about sleep hygiene, stress management and relaxation techniques which might bring positive well-being for mental health.
- Finally, menopause and emotion are very sensitive mental health issues and a kind of mystery so it is clear that emotional status based on surroundings psychosocial aspects of menopause management requires further research to bring more light on this issue.

REFERENCES

1. Desai HD, Jann MW. Major depression in women: a review of the literature. J Am Pharm Assoc (Wash). 2001;40:525-37.
2. Parry BL, Newton RP. Chronobiological basis of female-specific mood disorders. Neuropsychopharmacology. 2001;25(Suppl 5):S102-8.
3. Andrews G, Hall W, Teeson M, Henderson S. The Mental Health of Australia. Canberra: Commonwealth Department of Health and Aged Care; 1999.
4. Kornstein SG. The evaluation and management of depression in women across the life-span. J Clin Psychiatry. 2001;62(Suppl 24):11-7.
5. Robinson GE. Psychotic and mood disorders associated with the perimenopausal period: epidemiology, aetiology and management. CNS Drugs. 2001;15:1175-84.
6. Bourne EJ. The Anxiety and Phobia Workbook. California: New Harbinger Associations; 1995.
7. Walters CA. The psychosocial meaning of menopause: women's experiences. J Women Ageing. 2000;12:117-31.
8. Kravitz HM, Ganz PA, Bromberger J, Powell LH, Sutton-Tyrrell K, Meyer PM. Sleep difficulty in women at midlife: a community survey of sleep and the menopausal transition. Menopause. 2003;10:19.
9. Freedman RR, Roehrs TA. Sleep disturbance in menopause. Menopause. 2007;14:826.
10. Juang KD, Wang SJ, Lu SR, Lee SJ, Fuh JL. Hot flashes are associated with psychological symptoms of anxiety and depression in peri- and post- but not premenopausal women. Maturitas. 2005;52:119.

11. Joffe H, Hall JE, Soares CN, Hennen J, Reilly CJ, Carlson K, et al. Vasomotor symptoms are associated with depression in perimenopausal women seeking primary care. Menopause. 2002;9:392.
12. Bonnet MH, Arand DL. Consequences of insomnia. Sleep Med Clin. 2006;1:351.
13. Vignola A, Lamoureux C, Bastien CH, Morin CM. Effects of chronic insomnia and use of benzodiazepines on daytime performance in older adults. J Gerontol B Psychol Sci Soc Sci. 2000;55:P54-62.
14. Lerner D, Amick BC 3rd, Rogers WH, Malspeis S, Bungay K, Cynn D. The Work Limitations Questionnaire. Med Care. 2001;39:72-85.
15. Breslau N, Roth T, Rosenthal L, Andreski P. Sleep disturbance and psychiatric disorders: a longitudinal epidemiological study of young adults. Biol Psychiatry. 1996;39:411.
16. Woznica AA, Carney CE, Kuo JR, Moss TG. The insomnia and suicide link: toward an enhanced understanding of this relationship. Sleep Med Rev. 2015;22:37.
17. Bonnet MH, Arand DL. Heart rate variability in insomniacs and matched normal sleepers. Psychosom Med. 1998;60:610.
18. Suka M, Yoshida K, Sugimori H. Persistent insomnia is a predictor of hypertension in Japanese male workers. J Occup Health. 2003;45:344.
19. Bonnet MH, Arand DL, Javaheri S. Cardiovascular implications of poor sleep. Sleep Med Clin. 2007;2:529.
20. Vgontzas AN, Liao D, Bixler EO, Chrousos GP, Vela-Bueno A. Insomnia with objective short sleep duration is associated with a high risk for hypertension. Sleep. 2009;32:491.
21. Bonnet MH, Burton GG, Arand DL. Physiological and medical findings in insomnia: implications for diagnosis and care. Sleep Med Rev. 2014;18:111.
22. Kalmbach DA, Pillai V, Arnedt JT, Drake CL. DSM-5 Insomnia and Short Sleep: Comorbidity Landscape and Racial Disparities. Sleep. 2016;39:2101.
23. Zheng B, Yu C, Lv J, Guo Y, Bian Z, Zhou M, et al. Insomnia symptoms and risk of cardiovascular diseases among 0.5 million adults: a 10-year cohort. Neurology. 2019;93:e2110.
24. Carter JR, Grimaldi D, Fonkoue IT, Medalie L, Mokhlesi B, Cauter EV, et al. Assessment of sympathetic neural activity in chronic insomnia: evidence for elevated cardiovascular risk. Sleep. 2018;41:48.
25. Fernandez-Mendoza J, He F, LaGrotte C, Vgontzas AN, Liao D, Bixler EO. Impact of the metabolic syndrome on mortality is modified by objective short sleep duration. J Am Heart Assoc. 2017;6:579.
26. Sherwin BB. Impact of the changing hormonal milieu on psychological functioning. In Lobo RA (Ed). Treatment of the Post-menopausal Woman: Basic and Clinical Aspects. New York: Raven Press; 1994. pp. 119-27.
27. Schmidt PJ, Nieman MD, Danaceau MA, Tobin MB, Roca CA, Murphy JH, et al. Estrogen replacement in perimenopause-related depression: a preliminary report. Am J Obstet Gynecol. 2000;183:414-20.
28. Soares CN, Almeida OP, Joffe H, Cohen LS. Efficacy of oestradiol for the treatment of depressive disorders in perimenopausal women: a double-blind, randomized, placebo-controlled trial. Arch Gen Psychiatry. 2001;58:529-34.

Premature Ovarian Insufficiency

CHAPTER 13

■ INTRODUCTION

Loss of ovarian function occurring in women younger than 40 years of age is called premature ovarian insufficiency (POI). It may be associated with intermittent resumption of ovarian activity in over 25% of women.[1]

Premature ovarian insufficiency may also be referred to as primary ovarian insufficiency, premature menopause, or premature/primary ovarian failure.

Fuller Albright,[2] a Harvard endocrinologist, first described the condition as primary ovarian insufficiency to indicate that the "primary" defect was within the ovary, but later it was found that ovarian insufficiency might occur from secondary causes. Although many still refer to it as primary ovarian insufficiency, or premature ovarian failure (POF), and premature menopause. The term "premature ovarian insufficiency" is recommended because "premature" encompasses both spontaneous and iatrogenic conditions, and "insufficiency," rather than failure, reflects the possibility of some intermittent ovarian activity and it may not be the total failure.

Premature ovarian insufficiency could be associated with ovulation and may result in pregnancy.

Because of long-term complications, POI is regarded as major public health issue. Also, there is an increasing numbers of young women surviving following cancer treatments, who will live the whole of their lives with iatrogenic POI. Given all these serious health issues, POI should be a public health priority so that they need to be supported and health-care professionals are given adequate education and resources to identify, manage POI at the earliest possible stage.

Diagnosis of POI often has long-term physical and psychological effect for women, so women may need emotional support and ongoing medical follow-up and repeated counseling.

■ PATHOLOGY

Ovaries are unresponsive to endogenous and exogenous follicle-stimulating hormone (FSH) due to genetic or immunological inactivation of the FSH or luteinizing hormone (LH) receptor (*see* genetic factors section).[3] It is also possible that spontaneous POI may occur as part of an aging syndrome in some women. There is increasing evidence that epigenetic aging can begin as early as a few weeks postconception in fetal tissues.[4]

EPIDEMIOLOGY

Premature ovarian insufficiency occurs in approximately 1% of the population and POI can occur spontaneously affecting up to 4% of women and may vary with ethnicity.[5]

Webber et al. described incidence of POI:[5]
- 1:10,000 at the age of 18-25 years,
- 1:1000 in women aged 25-30 years
- 1:100 in the age range 35-40 years.

The frequency of POI with primary amenorrhea is 10-28% and in those with secondary amenorrhea 4-18%.[6] A recent global prevalence study of POI and early menopause concluded that the pooled prevalence of POI was as high as 3.7% [95% confidence interval (CI) 3.1-4.3] and that the prevalence was higher in countries with a medium or low Human Development Index.[7]

Menopause occurring between 40 and 45 years of age is called early menopause, with spontaneous early menopause affecting approximately nearly 12% of women. "Resistant ovary syndrome" is a rare disorder characterized by elevated levels of FSH and LH despite normal anti-Müllerian hormone (AMH) and antral follicle count (AFC). The ovaries are unresponsive to endogenous and exogenous FSH. It is different from POI. Resistant ovaries occur due to genetic or immunological inactivation of the FSH or LH receptors.[3] Early ovarian insufficiency or early menopause is difficult to predict. Sometimes in the lead-up, the time between periods becomes longer or erratic. However, there is no specific menstrual pattern which signals that early menopause is about to occur. POI women suffer from estrogen deficiency. So women with POI complains of hot flushes, mood changes, sleep disturbance, vaginal dryness, or poor lubrication during sexual arousal. These symptoms may occur even while the woman is still having menstrual periods. The onset of symptoms may occur gradually or suddenly especially after surgical menopause. Symptoms may be more severe in comparison to women experiencing natural menopause.

When women came to know the diagnosis of POI, they start suffering from severe emotional turmoil. Women often feel confused, sad, or jealous of other women's pregnancies or get old before their time. Depression and anxiety are commonly experienced. Psychological counseling can ease this distress. Use of menopausal hormone therapy (MHT), also known as hormone replacement therapy (HRT), may help her. Support from the woman's partner, family, and a friend is important.

ETIOLOGY AND PATHOGENESIS

The etiology is unknown in 70-90% of diagnosed women.[8] Pathogenesis is not fully understood what causes this condition and how to optimally manage the many squeals of a premature cessation of ovarian activity resulting in a chronic hypoestrogenic state.[9,10]

Premature ovarian insufficiency may occur as a part of an aging syndrome in some women, evidence that epigenetic aging can begin as early as a few weeks postconception in fetal tissues.[4]

The other causes include genetic (X chromosome-related and autosomal), more genetic mutations have recently been discovered by whole-genome sequences.[11]

Turner syndrome, Fragile X syndrome, also autosomal mutations.

Metabolic Causes

- The autosomal genetic defect known as galactosemia.
- Autoimmune Hashimoto's thyroiditis, type I diabetes, adrenal insufficiency, Sjögren's syndrome, rheumatoid arthritis, inflammatory bowel disease, multiple sclerosis, celiac disease, and myasthenia gravis.
- Infectious mumps[12] or human immunodeficiency virus, either due to antiviral medications or the virus,[13] as well as possibly tuberculosis, malaria, cytomegalovirus, and varicella.
- Metabolic, toxin-related, and iatrogenic including following chemotherapy, radiation, or surgery[14,15] (uterine artery embolization and pelvic surgery, including treatment of torsions, endometriomas, ovarian cysts, and pelvic malignancies, or electively for genetic BRCA carriers, may also be responsible).

Toxic Cause

Premature ovarian insufficiency has been associated with polycyclic aromatic hydrocarbon exposure, e.g., in cigarette smoke.[16-18]

Iatrogenic Causes

Premature ovarian insufficiency can occur as a result of chemotherapy, radiation, or surgical therapies. The effects of chemotherapy depend on the type, previous ovarian reserve, dosage, and age at administration.[19,20]

■ DIAGNOSIS OF PREMATURE OVARIAN INSUFFICIENCY

History-taking

Diagnosis and evaluation of POI, apart from karyotype, cover exclusion of other conditions leading to amenorrhea, such as pregnancy, thyroid gland diseases, or hyperprolactinemia. An important part of the evaluation is the assessment of the possibility of autoimmune diseases that may accompany POF.

It is important to take a careful personal and family history of the following:
- Genetic abnormalities
- Family history of premature or early menopause
- Early menarche
- Nulliparity/low parity

- Cigarette smoking (dose-response effect)
- Underweight.

The presentation of POI is usually one of secondary amenorrhea or oligomenorrhea, subfertility, and estrogen deficiency symptoms. However, the spontaneous POI phenotype can be extremely variable, with some women presenting with few or no symptoms apart from variable degrees of amenorrhea. Multiple factors influence symptoms including the cause of POI; symptoms may be more severe and may differ qualitatively (e.g., psychosocially/psychosexually in iatrogenic POI).[21-23] Symptoms may also be more severe in POI than those experienced with menopause at the natural age.[21]

Investigation: Biochemical Markers

Premature ovarian insufficiency can be confirmed by two elevated FSH tests, 4–6 weeks apart[24] is >40 IU/L, although the National Institute for Health and Care Excellence guideline suggests >30 IU/L[25] and the European Society of Human Reproduction and Embryology guideline suggests a lower cut-off of >25 IU/L.[25]

If there is still some menstruation, these tests should be performed on days 2–3 of the cycle. It is important, however, that POI is not overdiagnosed in those with regular cycles and no history of relevant menstrual disturbance.

Anti-Müllerian hormone should not be routinely used to diagnose POI, but may have a role when the diagnosis of POI is inconclusive. POI will be expected to have low-serum AMH.[26]

An AMH test could be performed to support the diagnosis of POI, problems with assay sensitivity/reliability prevent routine use currently.[1]

Although no diagnostic cut-off is established and AMH can be undetectable for as long as 5 years before periods cease; additionally, lack of universal availability, especially in primary care, and cost preclude this from being used routinely as a diagnostic test for POI.[25]

Serum urea, electrolytes, and creatinine (UEC), comprehensive metabolic panel (CMP), liver function test (LFT), thyroid-stimulating hormone (TSH), 25-hydroxy vitamin D. Bone turnover markers: not currently recommended for routine use. But when reduced bone mass is present, we need to consider the following: serum parathyroid hormone (PTH), celiac serology, and 24-hour urine calcium excretion.

Imaging DXA (dual-energy X-ray absorptiometry): Indicated at initial diagnosis for all women with POI, "Low bone mass" (Z score <−2) is the preferred term instead of osteopenia in this setting. T scores <−2.5 may be used to define osteoporosis.[26]

Plain imaging: Vertebral fracture assessment should be considered on an individual basis, particularly if concerns regarding height loss, back pain, chronic diseases associated with low bone mineral density (BMD) and current or past glucocorticoid use. Whole-genome sequencing might enable identification of novel causative genomic factors not yet identified by targeted gene sequencing.

For spontaneous POI, assessment of the karyotype and the FMR1 gene premutation should be offered.

Where resources are limited, women with early POI (<30 years old), those with learning difficulties, and those with a family history of POI can be prioritized for genetic testing, although ideally all women with POI would be offered this. 2.5-20% of women with POI have evidence of adrenal autoimmunity with histological evidence of autoimmune oophoritis, and 10-20% of patients with Addison's disease have POI.[27]

Testing for adrenal cortex or 21-hydroxylase antibodies in peripheral blood is the most sensitive test and should be screened for in all POI patients. If positive, adrenal function tests should then be performed. Thyroid peroxidase, autoantibodies, baseline DXA bone densitometry, and the change in BMD with time (*see* "Bone health" section).

The early hormonal deprivation contributes to the impairment of central and peripheral components of the sexual response, resulting in hypoactive sexual desire disorder (HSDD) and symptomatic vulvovaginal atrophy (VVA)/genitourinary syndrome of menopause (GSM).[28] Vaginal maturation index or testosterone estimation can be done if it is indicated. Women suffer much distress once she knows the diagnosis. Significant emotional and cognitive "rebuilding" is required due to the multiple effects of POI including infertility, potential early aging, and reduced self-esteem.[29]

In women with POI, lower androgen levels alone do not account for the amount of sexual dysfunction and the poor sense of well-being and sexual satisfaction.[30] Some more tests may be required to differentiate the diagnosis.

Cardiometabolic health may be compromised in women with POI. It is now well-recognized that POI is associated with an increased incidence of cardiovascular and cerebrovascular disease. Even basal FSH levels >7 IU/L have been found to be associated with adverse cardiovascular risk marker changes.[31]

Tao et al. detected a 48% higher risk of ischemic heart disease in POI, compared to the risk in women whose last menstruation was at 50 years of age. POI is an independent risk factor for ischemic heart disease and coronary vascular disease,[32] therefore in suspected cases we may need to do electrocardiogram (ECG) and echocardiogram.

Compared with women who had menopause at 50-51 years, the risk of cardiovascular disease (CVD) (coronary heart disease or stroke) was greater in women with POI [hazard ratio (HR) 1.55, 95% CI 1.38-1.73; p <0.0001].

Finally, gist for diagnosis of premature ovarian insufficiency.

Full history, e.g., menstrual health, is important in making the diagnosis. The diagnosis should not be made on the basis of only one FSH level. AMH testing is only required if there is diagnostic uncertainty. Investigations of karyotype, fragile X and adrenal antibody status are recommended for spontaneous POI. A baseline DXA scan should be offered to all women diagnosed with POI.

Treatments

General

Women who are diagnosed with POI should be advised to observe a well-balanced diet with adequate exercise and maintain a healthy weight range, whilst avoiding smoking and minimizing alcohol consumption. Women should be advised to maintain healthy lifestyle by:

- Weight-bearing exercise
- Avoidance of smoking
- Maintenance of normal body weight
- Balanced diet containing the recommended intake of calcium and vitamin D—dietary supplements may be required if inadequate intake
- Avoiding excess alcohol.

Women with primary ovarian insufficiency should be encouraged to maintain a lifestyle that optimizes bone and cardiovascular health, including engaging in regular weight-bearing exercise, maintaining an adequate intake of calcium (1,200 mg daily) and vitamin D (at least 800 IU daily), eating a healthy diet to avoid obesity, and undergoing screening for cardiovascular risk factors, with treatment of any identified risk factors.

These approaches, combined with adequate MHT, should reduce the risk of CVD and osteoporosis, although specific clinical trial evidence is lacking. The benefits of early initiation of MHT have been confirmed in many recent trials and meta-analyses of naturally and surgically menopausal women. The dose and type of hormones at initiation of therapy appear crucial for coronary heart disease benefits,[33] so if necessary, full cardiac evaluation could be done before starting MHT.

Premature ovarian insufficiency has a multisystem impact with profound physical and emotional ramifications; MHT at least until the average age of menopause should be first-line treatment unless contraindicated or if rejected by the woman after careful counseling.

Appropriate HRT to replace premenopausal levels of ovarian sex steroids is paramount to increase the quality-of-life for women with POI and ameliorate the associated health risks. Also, its management should be done by multidisciplinary teams or with multiprofessional collaboration.

Principles of hormone therapy (HT) in POI are to resume or restoring the physiological hormonal environment as closely as possible to natural milieu. This environment will achieve the most optimal health outcomes in POI

(maximizing benefits and minimizing side effects/risks). As MHT needs to be used for long time, the principles of MHT should be like:
- The hormones replaced should be identical to those which are missing.
- Nonoral estrogen delivery routes may be chosen if possible. As nonoral estrogen gets the advantages in regard to avoiding first-pass hepatic metabolism and thus minimizing the prothrombotic effect of oral estrogen.
- Estrogen-containing hormone as estrogen reduces insulin sensitivity, low-density lipoprotein (LDL), thickness of media, intima, increases sex hormone-binding globulin (SHBG), release nitric oxide (NO), and reduces oxidative stress and angiotensin enzyme convertor.
- Lower doses of MHT may be used initially to assess tolerance or any side effects but higher doses of estradiol are usually required in POI.

A typical "physiological" estrogen regimen might consist of estradiol 75-100 µg patches or three to four metered 0.75 mg doses of estrogel. Oral estradiol (2-4 mg/day) can be safely used in nonobese women thought not to be at increased risk of thrombosis. These doses achieve relatively physiological levels of estradiol of 200-400 pmol/L. The rationale for recommending higher doses of HT is that, as well as symptom relief, there appears to be a dose-response effect regarding cardiovascular and bone benefits, although there are few dose-response trials of HT in POI having good effects too.[34]

Observational data have shown that women with POI have a lower risk of breast cancer compared with controls. HRT does not appear to increase the risk of breast cancer in younger menopausal women under the age of 50 years.

There is limited evidence on the risk of venous thromboembolism (VTE) in women with POI or that associated with the use of sex steroid hormone replacement. Data from large observational studies and meta-analyses have shown that transdermal administration of estradiol is unlikely to increase the risk of VTE in naturally menopausal women. The transdermal route of estradiol administration should therefore be considered in women with POI who are at increased risk of venous thrombosis including those with raised body mass index. Women with POI can switch to no-bleed continuous combined regimens after a couple of years if they wish, or start immediately if they have presented with >1 year amenorrhea. Although continuous combined HT is associated with greater endometrial safety.[35]

Progesterone/progestogens: A "physiological" endometrial protection regimen in nonhysterectomized women can be achieved with 200 mg micronized progesterone administered orally or vaginally for 12 days per cycle. 200 microgram micronized progesterone in combined HT is natural progesterone. The metabolic benefits of estrogen are maintained, by the combination with micronized progesterone and is not prothrombotic and there appears to be a lower risk of breast cancer in natural menopause.[36]

Studies clearly showed that women receiving shorter courses or no HT have a greater risk of cardiovascular, bone, and cognitive pathology and the considerable benefits of HT used in POI for quality-of-life, bone, cardiovascular, and cognitive health, the pros usually far outweigh the cons for HT to be used long term, at least until the average age of menopause.

Duration of treatment Advisory guidelines 25 NICE Guideline [NG23]: Menopause diagnosis and management. https://www.nice.org.uk/guidance/ng23. [Last accessed March 2021].

International Menopause Society (IMS) recommends that treatment of POI with MHT should continue at least until the average age of menopause (51 years).

Until this age, this constitutes genuine replacement of hormones, which would have naturally been produced if the ovaries were working normally, in contrast to replacement following natural menopause **(Fig. 1)**. A recent Global Consensus Statement[37] coordinated by the IMS, formulated mainly from a systematic review and meta-analysis of all the relevant randomized controlled trial (RCT) data, concluded that naturally and surgically menopausal women receiving physiological doses of testosterone could achieve a significant improvement in sexual desire without any adverse effects apart from excess hair growth or acne.

There is increasing evidence that women with POI have lower androgen levels compared to age-matched controls. This might have an adverse effect on sexual desire, arousal, and orgasm and may contribute to other health problems such as tiredness, loss of stamina, osteopenia, and sarcopenia. A systematic review and meta-analysis of testosterone levels performed in different types of spontaneous POI included 529 women compared to 319 controls showed in addition to estrogen and progesterone/progestogen therapy, women with POI may benefit from androgen replacement.[38]

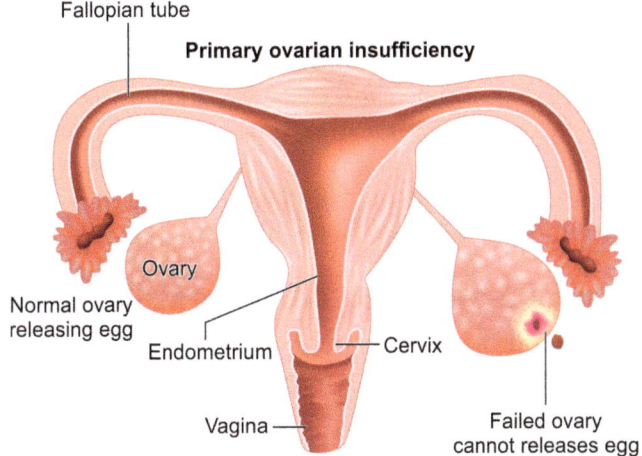

Fig. 1: Premature ovarian failure.

The problem is the global lack of license of testosterone for female treatment, options to achieve the required physiological dose of 5 mg/day (compared to 50 mg/day in men). The consensus concluded that there were insufficient data to make a recommendation for the use of oral dehydroepiandrosterone (DHEA) to improve female sexual desire.[39]

The risk of breast cancer with long-term MHT usage in POI is not thought to be any higher than that of the age-matched non-POI population.[40]

■ PREVENTION OF BONE LOSS

Osteoporosis is a key concern for women with POI.[22,23] Prevalence of osteoporosis is estimated as ranging from 8 to 27% according to the definition used (BMD or fracture). Women with POI have significantly lower BMD.[41] Osteoporosis is more common in women who have had estrogen deficiency since young age. All guidelines agreed that MHT should be initiated and continued until at least the age of usual menopause.[42] Assessment of BMD should be considered at the time of diagnosis of POI. The frequency of repeat bone density assessment should be guided by the woman's risk for developing osteoporosis and consideration should be given to repeat BMD assessment in women with osteoporosis within 2–3 years of the diagnosis. Management of women with POI where MHT is contraindicated, such as women with breast cancer, requires specialist referral for consideration of alternative antiresorptive therapies, such as bisphosphonates or denosumab.

It is important to check BMD every 2 years, particularly if the woman decides against taking HRT as the use of HRT prevents bone loss. A healthy lifestyle is important to maintain bone health. They should avoid smoking, engage in regular weight-bearing exercise, and ensure adequate dietary intake of calcium and vitamin D. If a woman suffers a bone fracture from osteoporosis, there are several proven therapies available to reduce her risk of further fractures. However, specialist consultation is recommended to consider future fertility requirements and impact of antiresorptive therapy (RCTs). Treatment with more "physiological" doses of 100–150 μg transdermal or 2 mg oral estradiol may be superior to 30 μg ethinylestradiol for spine BMD accrual and bone turnover marker response.[43,44] A decrease in BMD on subsequent scans (bone loss >5% and/or >0.05 g/cm^2) should prompt review of estrogen replacement therapy and of other potential factors. Development of a fragility fracture should prompt referral to an osteoporosis specialist.

■ GENITOURINARY SYNDROME OF MENOPAUSE

The early hormonal deprivation contributes to the impairment of central and peripheral components of the sexual response, resulting in HSDD and VVA/GSM.[32]

The absence of the vital effect of estrogens on sexual pathways[45] increases dyspareunia. Also, there is increased 2.8-fold increased risk of sexual dysfunction in women with POI.[46] However, systemic HT does not completely resolve sexual symptoms in women with POI.[47] Both estrogens and androgens cooperate in the brain and genitourinary physiology[48] so restoration of their deficiency should be strongly considered in the context of a biopsychosocial approach, for postmenopausal women. MHT may relieve hot flushes and/or night sweats and patient satisfaction. Combining elements of cognitive behavioral therapy with sexual health education are necessary. Local estrogen cream may be used. VVA symptoms can be very severe in young women following treatment for malignancy, particularly whilst using aromatase inhibitors after breast cancer. Even ultra-low-dose vaginal estrogen is contraindicated in women on aromatase inhibitors. Women with breast cancer on tamoxifen can use estrogen off-label due to blockage of estrogen receptors by tamoxifen.[49] Prasterone has not yet been sufficiently studied in women with a history of breast cancer or other malignancies to make specific recommendations.

Nonestrogenic VVA treatments include bioadhesive moisturizers that are hydrophilic and rehydrate vaginal tissues, providing a reasonable alternative to vaginal estrogen. They are a more physiological way of replacing vaginal secretions than vaginal gels/lubricants such as KY jelly. Lubricants and moisturizers should have similar osmolality and pH to those of physiological vaginal secretions.[50]

The consensus concluded that there were insufficient data to make a recommendation for the use of oral DHEA to improve female sexual desire.[51]

■ CONTRACEPTION

A diagnosis of POI does not exclude the possibility of ovarian activity and ovulation, with approximately a 5% chance of natural conception. Use of HT might actually increase the chance of pregnancy slightly through suppression of high FSH and LH levels, which may otherwise downregulate ovarian receptors and cause premature luteinization of follicles, thus facilitating ovulation of any remaining oocytes.[52,53]

It is therefore important that adequate contraception is used if pregnancy is not desired.

The combined oral contraceptive (COC) containing ethinylestradiol has been extensively used for puberty induction and HT in POI. The COC is generally cheap, easily accessible, familiar to women and health-care professionals, and provides contraception, if required. It is particularly popular with young women requiring hormonal support for POI.

Oral contraceptive pills can be used as a replacement hormone up to the age of 50 years if the woman has no contraindications to its use including risk factors or a personal history of venous blood clots, hypertension, or is a current smoker and older than 34 years. Continuous or extended cycle use of the oral contraceptive pill (OCP) is preferred as women may experience a return of symptoms when the inactive tablets are taken and to optimize bone health.[14]

When contraception is required or if there are vaginal bleeding problems, a levonorgestrel intrauterine system releasing 20 μg/day can be used in combination with transdermal or oral estrogen, which provides up to 5 years of endometrial protection. Levonorgestrel intrauterine system protects endometrial hyperplasia even with higher doses of estrogen is used.

Eventually, the COC regimen can be switched to MHT when the risk of unwanted pregnancy is highly unlikely, typically >2 years postdiagnosis.

■ PREVENTION OF CARDIOVASCULAR DISEASE

Premature ovarian insufficiency is associated with an increased risk of CVD. Some studies suggest that this risk is minimized in women who take HRT.

Women with early menopause should minimize CVD risk by maintaining normal weight, exercising regularly, ceasing smoking, maintaining a healthy diet, controlling diabetes mellitus and high blood pressure, and preventing or treating high levels of cholesterol and triglycerides. Each year of increased risk of CVD.[54] The benefits of early initiation of HT analyses in naturally and surgically menopausal women have been confirmed in many recent trials[12] and meta-analysis. The dose and type of hormones at initiation of therapy appear crucial for coronary heart disease benefits.[33]

In women with POI, meta-analyses have shown that those who used HT for longer, especially greater than 10 years, have the lowest risk of CVD when compared with women who do not use HT.[55] Cardiovascular outcomes appear to vary according to the type of estrogen used.

Women with POI were randomized to either transdermal estradiol with oral progesterone, or to a 30 μg ethinylestradiol COC. Mean systolic blood pressure (between-group difference 7.3 mm Hg, 95% CI 2.5-12.00 mm Hg) and diastolic (7.4 mm Hg, 95% CI 2.5-12.00 mm Hg) blood pressure, plasma angiotensin II, and serum creatinine were significantly lower in the HT group than in the COC group at the end of the 12-month treatment.[56]

■ FERTILITY ISSUES

Involuntary childlessness is one of the most significant consequences for women diagnosed with POI. Not only may this adversely affect her psychological well-being but, worldwide, it may compromise a woman's status in her community and impact her economic stability and empowerment.

There is still a low chance (1-5% over a lifetime) of becoming pregnant spontaneously (unless a woman has had an oophorectomy), so if a woman does not want a pregnancy, she should use contraception even if diagnosed with POI.

Some women may choose not to become a parent, others may want to adopt or foster children.

Some women may try in vitro fertilization (IVF) or drugs to stimulate egg production but these have a low chance of success than women without POI.

Most women with POI who achieve pregnancy use eggs from another woman donated either anonymously or by a friend or relative. Another option is achieving pregnancy by using embryos donated by another couple.

Stem cell therapies, platelet-rich plasma, and primordial follicle activation all require further research and confirmation of efficacy and safety before routine recommendation.

From Rejuvenation to Ovarian Rescue

Although it is popularly known as "ovarian rejuvenation," in actual fact, this procedure consists of rescuing follicles that were already in that ovary, so it would be more appropriate to call it "ovarian rescue." This technique does not rejuvenate, but rather it recovers the dormant/sleeping follicles. The stem cells activate this ovarian niche in order to rescue the follicles that are already there, so that they grow and mature to finally provide mature eggs for the patients.

The ASCOT technique (involving infusion of stem cells in the ovarian artery), which has recently been shown to be successful in low-responder patients, has now shown that it can achieve pregnancy in a woman with POF.[57]

Cryopreservation and transplantation may be carefully considered before cancer treatment in order to preserve endocrine function and fertility in young patients with cancer.[58]

More research is needed to determine whether these approaches are realistic paradigm in the management of older women with depleted ovarian reserve.

■ COMPLEMENTARY THERAPIES

There are no good data for the use of complementary therapies in POI; HT should be first-line treatment unless there are specific contraindications or according to the woman's wishes, having made an evidence-based decision after being fully counseled.

■ PHARMACOLOGICAL ALTERNATIVES

Nonhormonal pharmacological options (e.g., paroxetine, venlafaxine, gabapentin, oxybutynin, and clonidine) should only be advised for the alleviation of vasomotor symptoms where HT is contraindicated—for example, hormone receptor-positive breast cancer or if the individual wishes to avoid HT despite adequate counseling on risks and benefits.[59]

Preventive measures such as optimizing lifestyle, diet and exercise, and advice regarding long-term hormone replacement for this endocrine deficiency disorder, at least until the age of natural menopause, will have the greatest impact on the quality-of-life of women with POI.

KEY MESSAGES

- Premature ovarian insufficiency is characterized by cessation of menstruation and decline in ovarian function before the age of 40 years. It is a concerning condition for many reasons.
- Women with spontaneous and surgical POI suffers from subfertility and is at significantly greater risk of CVD, bone loss, cognitive and psychosexual disorder, and other chronic conditions.
- Confirmation of the elevated FSH level and a low estradiol level would confirm the diagnosis of primary ovarian insufficiency. This information is a highly emotional and sensitive issue.
- They need to be counseled very delicately. Patients should understand that remission may occur and even pregnancy may happen, though unlikely, in 5–10% of cases.
- A karyotype analysis, tests for the FMR1 premutation and adrenal autoimmunity, a pelvic ultrasound examination, and measurement of BMD are indicated at the time of diagnosis.
- Optimizing lifestyle, diet and exercise, and advice regarding long-term hormone replacement MHT, at least until the age of natural menopause, will have the greatest impact if instituted at the earliest stage.
- There are very few data for the benefits and risks of complementary and alternative medicines and nonhormonal bone-sparing agents in POI.
- Replacement can be with the COC initially, if contraception is required, but in the long-term, MHT is recommended to optimize bone and metabolic health.
- Registration and research need to be carried out with POI.
- Recent advances in options such as IVM (in vitro maturation) and stem cell therapy, autologous mitochondrial transfer, stem cell-based neogenesis, and artificial gametes likely to be the future of treatment and may generate new hope for these patients. Donor egg/embryo is usually required to achieve a pregnancy.
- Premature ovarian insufficiency needs holistic tender and empathetic approach involving multidisciplinary collaboration to optimize the best outcome.

REFERENCES

1. Bachelot A, Nicolas C, Bidet M, Dulon J, Leban M, Golmard JL, et al. Long-term outcome of ovarian function in women with intermittent premature ovarian insufficiency. Clin Endocrinol (Oxf). 2017;86(2):223-8.
2. Albright F, Smith PH, Fraser R. A syndrome characterized by primary ovarian insufficiency and decreased stature: report of 11 cases with a digression on hormonal control of axillary and pubic hair. Am J Med Sci. 1942;204:625-48.
3. Huhtaniemi I, Alevizaki M. Gonadotrophin resistance. Best Pract Res Clin Endocrinol Metab. 2006;20(4):561-76.
4. Hoshino A, Horvath S, Sridhar A, Chitsazan A, Reh TA. Synchrony and asynchrony between an epigenetic clock and developmental timing. Sci Rep. 2019;9:3770.

5. Webber L, Davies M, Anderson R, Bartlett J, Braat D, et al. European Society for Human Reproduction and Embryology (ESHRE) Guideline Group on POI; ESHRE guideline: management of women with premature ovarian insufficiency. Hum Reprod. 2016;31(5):926-37.
6. Anasti JN. Premature ovarian failure: an update. Fertil Steril. 1998;70(1):1-15.
7. Golezar S, Ramezani Tehrani F, Khazaei S, Ebadi A, Keshavarz Z. The global prevalence of primary ovarian insufficiency and early menopause: a meta-analysis. Climacteric. 2019;22(4):403-11.
8. Maclaran K, Panay N. Premature ovarian failure. J Fam Plann Reprod Health Care. 2011;37(1):35-42.
9. Bricaire L, Odou MF, Cardot-Bauters C, Delemer B, North MO, Salenave S, et al. Frequent large germline HRPT2 deletions in a French National cohort of patients with primary hyperparathyroidism. J Clin Endocrinol Metab. 2013;98(2):E403-8.
10. Webber AL, Wood JM, Thompson B. Fine motor skills of children with amblyopia improve following binocular treatment. 2016;57(11):4713-20.
11. Heddar A, Dessen P, Flatters D, Misrahi M. Novel STAG3 mutations in a Caucasian family with primary ovarian insufficiency. Mol Genet Genomics. 2019;294:1527-34.
12. Van Kasteren YM, Hundscheid RD, Smits AP, Cremers FP, van Zonneveld P, Braat DD. Familial idiopathic premature ovarian failure: an overrated and underestimated genetic disease? Hum Reprod. 1999;14(10):2455-9.
13. Jiao X, Qin C, Li J, Qin Y, Gao X, Zhang B, et al. Cytogenetic analysis of 531 Chinese women with premature ovarian failure. Hum Reprod. 2012;27(7):2201-7.
14. Hernandez-Angeles C, Castelo-Branco C. Early menopause: a hazard to a woman's health. Indian J Med Res. 2016;143(4):420-7.
15. Overbeek A, van den Berg MH, van Leeuwen FE, Kaspers GJL, Lambalk CB, van Dulmen-den Broeder E. Chemotherapy-related late adverse effects on ovarian function in female survivors of childhood and young adult cancer: a systematic review. Cancer Treat Rev. 2017;53:10-24.
16. Vabre P, Gatimel N, Moreau J, Gayrard V, Picard-Hagen N, Parinau J, et al. Environmental pollutants, a possible etiology for premature ovarian insufficiency: a narrative review of animal and human data. Environ Health. 2017;16(1):37.
17. Ebrahimi M, Akbari Asbagh F. Pathogenesis and causes of premature ovarian failure: an update. Int J Fertil Steril. 2011;5(2):54-65.
18. Willett W, Stampfer MJ, Bain C, Lipnick R, Speizer FE, Rosner B, et al. Cigarette smoking, relative weight and menopause. Am J Epidemiol. 1983;117(6):651-8.
19. Oktem O, Okay K. Quantitative assessment of the impact of chemotherapy on ovarian follicle reserve and stromal function. Cancer. 2007;110(10):2222-9.
20. Spears N, Lopes F, Stefansdottir A, Rossi V, De Felici M, Anderson RA, et al. Ovarian damage from chemotherapy and current approaches to its protection. Hum Reprod Update. 2019;25(6):673-93.
21. Howard-Anderson J, Ganz PA, Bower JE, Stanton AL. Quality of life, fertility concerns, and behavioral health outcomes in younger breast cancer survivors: a systematic review. J Natl Cancer Inst. 2012;104(5):386-405.
22. Deeks AA, Gibson-Helm M, Teede H, Vincent A. Premature menopause: a comprehensive understanding of psychosocial aspects. Climacteric. 2011;14(5):565-72.
23. Singer D, Mann E, Hunter MS, Pitkin J, Panay N. The silent grief: psychosocial aspects of premature ovarian failure. Climacteric. 2011;14(4):428-37.
24. Baber RJ, Panay N, Fenton A; IMS Writing Group. 2016 IMS Recommendations on women's midlife health and menopause hormone therapy. Climacteric. 2016;19(2):109-50.
25. NICE Guideline [NG23]. Menopause diagnosis and management. [online] Available from: https://www.nice.org.uk/guidance/ng23. [Last accessed March 2021].

26. Nyström A, Mörse H, Nordlöf H, Wiebe K, Artman M, Øra I, et al. Anti-Müllerian hormone compared with other ovarian markers after childhood cancer treatment. Acta Oncol. 2019;58(2):218-24.
27. Kirshenbaum M, Orvieto R. Premature ovarian insufficiency (POI) and autoimmunity-an update appraisal. J Assist Reprod Genet. 2019;36(11):2207-15.
28. Nappi RE, Cucinella L, Martini E, Rossi M, Tiranini L, Martella S, et al. Sexuality in premature ovarian insufficiency. Climacteric. 2019;22(3):289-95.
29. Graziottin A. Menopause and sexuality: key issues in premature menopause and beyond. Ann NY Acad Sci. 2010;1205:254-61.
30. van der Stege JG, Groen H, van Zadelhoff SJ, Lambalk CB, Braat DDM, van Kasteren YM, et al. Decreased androgen concentrations and diminished general and sexual well-being in women with premature ovarian failure. Menopause. 2008;15(1):23-31.
31. Chu MC, Rath KM, Huie J, Taylor HS. Elevated basal FSH in normal cycling women is associated with unfavourable lipid levels and increased cardiovascular risk. Hum Reprod. 2003;18(8):1570-3.
32. Roeters van Lennep JE, Heida KV, Bots ML, Hoek A; collaborators of the Dutch Multidisciplinary Guideline Development Group on Cardiovascular Risk Management after Reproductive Disorders. Cardiovascular disease in women with premature ovarian insufficiency: a systematic review and meta-analysis. Eur J Prev Cardiol. 2016;23(2):178-86.
33. Gerval MO, Stevenson J. Establishing the risk related to hormone replacement therapy and cardiovascular disease in women. Clin Pharm. 2017;5:7-24.
34. Cleemann L, Holm K, Kobbernagel H, Kristensen B, Skouby SO, Jensen AK, et al. Dosage of estradiol, bone and body composition in Turner syndrome: a 5-year randomized controlled clinical trial. Eur J Endocrinol. 2017;176(2):233-42.
35. Furness S, Roberts H, Marjoribanks J, Lethaby A. Hormone therapy in postmenopausal women and risk of endometrial hyperplasia. Cochrane Database Syst Rev. 2012;(8):CD000402.
36. Panay N; Medical Advisory Council of the British Menopause Society. BMS - Consensus statement: Bioidentical HRT. Post Reprod Health. 2019;25(2):61-3.
37. Davis SR, Baber R, Panay N, Bitzer J, Perez SC, Islam RM, et al. Global Consensus Position Statement on the use of testosterone therapy for women. Climacteric. 2019;22(5):429-34.
38. Janse F, Tanahatoe SJ, Eijkemans MJ, Fauser BC. Testosterone concentrations, using different assays, in different types of ovarian insufficiency: a systematic review and meta- analysis. Hum Reprod Update. 2012;18(4):405-19.
39. Islam RM, Bell RJ, Green S, Page MJ, Davis SR. Safety and efficacy of testosterone for women: a systematic review and meta-analysis of randomised controlled trial data. Lancet Diabetes Endocrinol. 2019;7(10):754-66.
40. Wu X, Cai H, Kallianpur A, Li H, Yang G, Gao J, et al. Impact of premature ovarian failure on mortality and morbidity among Chinese women. PLoS One. 2014;9(3):e89597.
41. Gallagher JC. Effect of early menopause on bone mineral density and fractures. Menopause. 2007;14(3 Pt 2):567-71.
42. Vujovic S, Brincat M, Erel T, Gambacciani M, Lambrinoudaki I, Moen MH, et al. EMAS position statement: managing women with premature ovarian failure. Maturitas. 2010;67(1):91-3.
43. Crofton PM, Evans N, Bath LE, Warner P, Whitehead TJ, Critchley HO, et al. Physiological versus standard sex steroid replacement in young women with premature ovarian failure: effects on bone mass acquisition and turnover. Clin Endocrinol (Oxf). 2010;73(6):707-14.
44. Cartwright B, Robinson J, Seed PT, Fogelman I, Rymer J. Hormone replacement therapy versus the combined oral contraceptive pill in premature ovarian failure: a randomized controlled trial of the effects on bone mineral density. J Clin Endocrinol Metab. 2016;101(9):3497-505.

45. Nappi RE, Polatti F. The use of estrogen therapy in women's sexual functioning (CME). J Sex Med. 2009;6(3):603-16.
46. De Almeida DM, Benetti-Pinto CL, Makuch MY. Sexual function of women with premature ovarian failure. Menopause. 2011;18(3):262-6.
47. Pacello PC, Yela DA, Rabelo S, Giraldo PC, Benetti-Pinto CL. Dyspareunia and lubrication in premature ovarian failure using hormonal therapy and vaginal health. Climacteric. 2014;17(4):342-7.
48. Simon JA, Goldstein I, Kim NN, Davis SR, Kellogg-Spadt S, Lowenstein L, et al. The role of androgens in the treatment of genitourinary syndrome of menopause (GSM): International Society for the Study of Women's Sexual Health (ISSWSH) expert consensus panel review. Menopause. 2018;25(7):837-47.
49. Sturdee DW, Panay N; International Menopause Society Writing Group. Recommendations for the management of postmenopausal vaginal atrophy. Climacteric. 2010;13(6):509-22.
50. Edwards D, Panay N. Treating vulvovaginal atrophy/genitourinary syndrome of menopause: how important is vaginal lubricant and moisturizer composition? Climacteric. 2016;19(2):151-61.
51. Let's talk about sex (Editorial). Lancet Diabetes Endocrinol. 2019;7:754-66.
52. Ben-Nagi J, Panay N. Premature ovarian insufficiency: how to improve reproductive outcome? Climacteric. 2014;17(3):242-6.
53. Dragojević Dikić S, Vasiljević M, Jovanović A, Dikić S, Jurišić A, Srbinović L, et al. Premature ovarian insufficiency: novel hormonal approaches in optimizing fertility. Gynecol Endocrinol. 2020;36(2):162-5.
54. Zhu D, Chung HF, Dobson AJ, Pandeya N, Giles GG, Bruinsma F, et al. Age at natural menopause and risk of incident cardiovascular disease: a pooled analysis of individual patient data. Lancet Public Health. 2019;4(11):e553-64.
55. Tsiligiannis S, Panay N, Stevenson JC. Premature ovarian insufficiency and long-term health consequences. Curr Vasc Pharmacol. 2019;17(6):604-9.
56. Langrish JP, Mills NL, Bath LE, Warner P, Webb DJ, Kelnar CJ, et al. Cardiovascular effects of physiological and standard sex steroid replacement regimens in premature ovarian failure. Hypertension. 2009;53(5):805-11.
57. Pellicer De Castellvi N, Herraiz S, Romeu M, Martinez S, Buigues A, Gomez-Segui I, et al. Bone marrow derived stem cells restore ovarian function and fertility in premature ovarian insufficiency women. Interim report of a randomized trial: mobilization versus ovarian injection. In: Human Reproduction. Oxford OX2 6DP, England: Oxford University Press Great Clarendon St.; 2020.
58. Kim S, Lee Y, Lee S, Kim T. Ovarian tissue cryopreservation and transplantation in patients with cancer. Obstet Gynecol Sci. 2018;61(4):431-42.
59. Sassarini J, Lumsden MA. Non-hormonal management of vasomotor symptoms. Climacteric. 2013;16(Suppl 1):31-6.

Metabolic Syndrome and Menopause

CHAPTER 14

■ INTRODUCTION

Metabolic syndrome is defined as an assemblage of risk factors for cardiovascular diseases (CVD), the emergence of which is at high point in postmenopausal women. Metabolic syndrome is a multifactorial disease with multiple risk factors that arises from insulin resistance accompanying abnormal adipose deposition and function.[1,2] It comprises a combination of risk factors for coronary heart disease, as well as for diabetes, fatty liver, and several cancers. Metabolic disorders, metabolic syndrome (MetS), may occur in menopause which include dyslipidemia, disorders of carbohydrate metabolism [impaired glucose tolerance (IGT), type 2 diabetes mellitus (T2DM)], or components of metabolic syndrome, constitute risk factors for CVD in women. Menopause is associated with redistribution of body weight and weight gain in a majority of women. Weight gain and obesity largely drive the increased prevalence of metabolic syndrome in postmenopausal women.

The central features of the metabolic syndrome are insulin resistance, visceral adiposity, atherogenic dyslipidemia, and endothelial dysfunction. These conditions are interrelated and share common mediators, pathways, and pathophysiological mechanisms.

Physicians and scientists have long known that certain conditions increase a person's risk of developing atherosclerotic cardiovascular disease (ASCVD). These risk factors include a family history of premature coronary disease, hypertension, hyperlipidemia, diabetes, and smoking. Age both in male and female increases the risk of CVD, estrogen deficient state of postmenopausal women is another important risk factor for CVD. Of these risks, some can be modified—for example, cessation of smoking—whereas others, such as genetic predisposition, menopause cannot. The risk of CVD can be decreased by addressing these individual risk factors, both by lifestyle modifications and, if appropriate, pharmacologic treatment [National Cholesterol Education Program (NCEP), 2002].

The prevalence of MetS differs greatly in different populations. Among pre- and postmenopausal women it ranges from 13.8% to >60.0%.[3] Weight gain and obesity largely drive the increased prevalence of MetS in postmenopausal women.[4] Menopausal transition is associated with significant weight gain (2–2.5 kg over 3 years on average). Though menopause itself is not the main reason for weight gain.

IMPORTANCE

Each year 15 million people die from noncommunicable diseases between the age 3 and 69 years; over 85% of these premature death occur in low- and middle-income countries, Bangladesh is one of them (WHO 2018). The leading metabolic risk factors globally are elevated blood pressure (to which 19% deaths are attributed), followed by overweight and obesity and raised blood glucose.

The metabolic syndrome is a clustering of hyperglycemia, insulin resistance, obesity, and dyslipidemia. It is important for several reasons.

First, it identifies patients who are at high risk of developing atherosclerotic CVD and T2DM.

Second, by considering the relationships between the components of metabolic syndrome, we may be able to better understand the pathophysiology that links them with each other and with the increased risk of CVD.

Third, it facilitates epidemiological and clinical studies of pharmacological, lifestyle, and preventive treatment approaches.

The interesting finding is that the intervention that lower noncommunicable diseases risk factors can result in reducing premature death by half to two-thirds.

These are the controlling major risk factors such as harmful use of tobacco, alcohol consumption, obesity, unhealthy diet, physical activities and other healthy lifestyle during menopause transition are associated with the less subclinical atherosclerosis, highlighting the growing recognition that the midlife is a critical window for metabolic syndrome and cardiovascular prevention in women.

DEFINITION

The WHO definition was the first to tie together the key components of insulin resistance, obesity, dyslipidemia, and hypertension. The definition mandates that insulin resistance be present; without it, even if all the other criteria were met, the patient would not have metabolic syndrome. The WHO definition also allows patients with T2DM to be diagnosed with metabolic syndrome if they meet the other criteria. This definition is not easily applied clinically and does not lend itself as well to large epidemiologic studies, where rapid and simple assessment is important.

According to the NCEP ATP III (Adult Treatment Panel III) definition, metabolic syndrome is present if three or more of the following five criteria are met:

1. Waist circumference over 40″ (men) or 35″ (women).
2. Blood pressure over 130/85 mm Hg.
3. Fasting triglyceride (TG) level over 150 mg/dL.
4. Fasting high-density lipoprotein cholesterol (HDL-C) level <40 mg/dL (men) or 50 mg/dL (women).
5. Fasting blood sugar over 100 mg/dL.

The NCEP ATP III definition is one of the most widely used criteria of metabolic syndrome. It incorporates the key features of hyperglycemia/insulin resistance, visceral obesity, atherogenic dyslipidemia, and hypertension.

In 2005, the International Diabetes Foundation (IDF) published new criteria for metabolic syndrome (Zimmet et al., 2005). Although it includes the same general criteria as the other definitions, it requires obesity, but not necessarily insulin resistance, be present.

■ PATHOPHYSIOLOGY

It is determined by underlying metabolic syndrome; in fact, key role could be played here by hyperinsulinemia, insulin resistance, and visceral obesity, all contributing to dyslipidemia, oxidative stress, inflammation, alter coagulation, and atherosclerosis observed during the menopausal period.

Central features are: insulin resistance, visceral obesity, atherogenic dyslipidemia, and endothelial dysfunction. In patients with metabolic syndrome, weight loss can lead to improvements in multiple features at the same time, so a certain degree of adiposity appears to be required to manifest the abnormal pathophysiology. Conversely, there are patients who are obese but who do not manifest any of the other components of metabolic syndrome, so both metabolic predisposition to insulin resistance and obesity appear to be necessary for expression of the metabolic syndrome phenotype. Atherogenic dyslipidemia follows from insulin resistance and visceral obesity. Endothelial dysfunction also follows from insulin resistance and from adipokines and free fatty acids (FFAs) that are released from visceral adipose tissue. Both atherogenic dyslipidemia and endothelial dysfunction contribute mechanistically to the development of atherosclerosis and CVD.

Along with insulin resistance, visceral adiposity, atherogenic dyslipidemia, and endothelial dysfunction—findings such as systemic inflammation, hypercoagulability, or microalbuminuria are important to the pathophysiology.

■ OBESITY

After menopause the incidence of obesity increases, including visceral (android) obesity. Such fat distribution fosters the occurrence of a number of metabolic disorders, including fully manifested metabolic syndrome, and enhances the development of atherosclerosis. Toth et al. reported that postmenopausal women had greater amounts of whole body and intra-abdominal fat compared with premenopausal women.[5] The comparison of patients with normal BMI and those with high BMI showed that high BMI (>30 kg/m^2) had a significant negative effect on blood pressure (as evidenced by the increased frequency of hypertension in overweight and obese patients). It also negatively and significantly affected TG and fasting glucose levels, and that it was linked significantly to low levels of HDL-C, therefore with CVD risk factors.[6] Intra-abdominal fat cells produce a number of substances with an impact on inflammatory responses, insulin resistance, and an increased risk of CVDs. Some molecules, directly synthesized by adipocytes are called "adipokines." They control regulation of fat mass.[7] Furthermore, they can also exert a role in the control of blood pressure, lipoprotein metabolism, coagulation, immunity, and inflammation.[8,9] Menopausal women are characterized by elevated levels of leptin and resistin and decreased levels of adiponectin.

■ SIGNS AND SYMPTOMS

Clinical manifestations of metabolic syndrome include the following:
- Hypertension
- Hyperglycemia
- Hypertriglyceridemia
- Reduced high-density lipoprotein cholesterol
- Abdominal obesity
- *Chest pain or shortness of breath*: Suggesting the rise of cardiovascular and other complications
- *Acanthosis nigricans, hirsutism, peripheral neuropathy, and retinopathy*: In patients with insulin resistance and hyperglycemia or with diabetes mellitus
- *Xanthomas or xanthelasmas*: In patients with severe dyslipidemia.

■ DIAGNOSIS

National Cholesterol Education Program Adult Treatment Panel III of America has given guidelines for diagnosis of Metabolic syndrome in **Box 1**.

According to guidelines from the National Heart, Lung, and Blood Institute (NHLBI) and the American Heart Association (AHA), metabolic syndrome is diagnosed when a patient has at least three of the following five conditions:
1. Fasting glucose ≥ 100 mg/dL (or receiving drug therapy for hyperglycemia).
2. Blood pressure ≥ 130/85 mm Hg (or receiving drug therapy for hypertension).

BOX 1: National Cholesterol Education Program.

Adult Treatment Panel III (NCEP-ATP III)

Metabolic syndrome diagnosis suggested by the presence of three or more of the following features:

- Waist >35" in women (>31" in South Asians)
- Triglycerides >150 mg/dL (or on drug treatment with a fibrate or niacin for elevated TG)
- HDL-C <50 mg/dL (or on drug treatment with a fibrate or niacin for low HDL-C)
- SBP ≥130 or DBP ≥85 mm Hg (or on antihypertensive drug treatment)
- Fasting plasma glucose >100 mg/dL (or on drug treatment for elevated glucose)

(TG: triglycerides; DBP: diastolic blood pressure; HDL-C: high-density lipoprotein cholesterol; SBP: systolic blood pressure)

3. Triglycerides ≥ 150 mg/dL (or receiving drug therapy for hypertriglyceridemia).
4. HDL-C <40 mg/dL in men or <50 mg/dL in women (or receiving drug therapy for reduced HDL-C).
5. Waist circumference ≥ 102 cm (40″) in men or ≥88 cm (35″) in women; if Asian American ≥90 cm (35″) in men or ≥80 cm (32″) in women.

Initial laboratory studies in patients suspected of having metabolic syndrome should include standard chemistries to assess for hyperglycemia and renal dysfunction and lipid studies to assess for hypertriglyceridemia or low HDL levels.

If a family history of early coronary or other atherosclerotic disease in addition to HDL-C and low-density lipoprotein cholesterol (LDL-C), studies of lipoprotein(a), apolipoprotein-B100, high-sensitivity C-reactive protein (CRP), and [if the patient does not already merit the lowest LDL-C target (<70)], homocysteine and fractionated LDL-C.

In view of the various associations between metabolic syndrome and other conditions, additional helpful blood tests may include thyroid and liver studies, hemoglobin-A1c levels, and uric acid. Increased thyroid-stimulating hormone (TSH) has been linked to a higher prevalence of metabolic syndrome.[10] Hyperuricemia appears to be much more common in patients with metabolic syndrome than in the general population, and this is attributed to the inflammatory effects of metabolic syndrome.[11] Further studies should be pursued as clinical findings dictate.

Imaging Studies

Imaging studies are not routinely indicated in the diagnosis of metabolic syndrome. However, they may be appropriate for patients with symptoms or signs of the many complications of the syndrome. Complaints of chest pain, dyspnea, or claudication may warrant additional testing with electrocardiography (rest/stress ECG), ultrasonography (vascular or rest/stress echocardiography).

■ TREATMENT APPROACH

Whenever menopause women attend for any symptoms healthcare providers need to take detailed history and assess for metabolic syndrome if they are obese. Undiagnosed and untreated, metabolic disorders may adversely affect the length and quality of women's life. Prevention and treatment preceded by early diagnosis should be the main goal for the physicians involved in menopausal care.

The initial management of metabolic syndrome involves lifestyle modifications including changes in diet and exercise habits.[12] Indeed, evidence exists to support the notion that the diet, exercise, and pharmacologic interventions may inhibit the progression of metabolic syndrome to diabetes mellitus (**Box 2**).[13]

> **BOX 2:** Therapeutic lifestyle modification.
> - Specific contract with patient for goals and self-monitoring
> - Exercise—at least 30 minutes of moderate to vigorous physical activity on most days of the week. Using pedometer, walking >10,000 steps/day is desirable
> - Diet—reduction of weight by 7–10% over 1 year with reduced caloric intake and reduced consumption of simple carbohydrates (low glycemic index diet). Women should consume a diet rich in fruits and vegetables; whole-grain, high-fiber foods; limited intake of saturated fat to 10% of energy (if possible to 7%); cholesterol to 300 mg/d; no more than 1 alcoholic drink per day; consumption of trans-fatty acid (FA) should be as low as possible
> - Increased omega-3 FA consumption (~850–1000 mg EPA + DHA/day)
> - Women should not smoke and should avoid environmental tobacco smoke

(EPA: eicosapentaenoic acid; DHA: docosahexaenoic acid)

Treatment of hypertension had been based according to 2014 report of the Eighth Joint National Committee (JNC-8) has led to less stringent recommendations for drug therapy (140/90 mm Hg for most populations, 150/90 mm Hg for patients aged 60 years or older),[14] with continued emphasis on the importance of promoting healthy diet and exercise behaviors, as addressed by 2013 guidelines from the American College of Cardiology.[15,16] Nevertheless, more recent study data continue to support a more aggressive blood pressure goal of 120/80 mm Hg.

Surgical Considerations

At present, no surgical interventions for metabolic syndrome have been widely accepted. However, trials of bariatric surgery in patients who were morbidly obese and had metabolic syndrome suggested beneficial results including decreased insulin resistance and lower levels of inflammatory cytokines.[17]

Importantly, metabolic syndrome raises specific perioperative issues that should be considered in patients with metabolic syndrome undergoing any major surgical procedure.[18]

■ REFERRAL CONSULTATION

Consultations

Patients with diabetes should be referred to a diabetic nutritionist, if not an endocrinologist must be consulted. Patients with cardiac symptoms (chest pain, shortness of breath, palpitations) or an abnormal stress test may merit referral to a cardiologist. Referral to be done to a preventive cardiologist for primary or secondary prevention of CVD in these high-risk patients. Consultation with a sleep specialist is indicated if there are symptoms suggestive of sleep apnea, such as excessive fatigue or daytime somnolence, a history of snoring and witnessed apneas, or physical signs of untreated apnea such as resistant hypertension.

Patients who are at high risk for obesity-associated morbidity and mortality with a BMI > 40 kg/m^2 or with a BMI > 35 kg/m^2 plus 1 or more significant comorbid conditions may be referred for consideration of bariatric surgery when less invasive methods of weight loss have failed.

■ COMPLEMENTARY AND ALTERNATIVE MEDICINE

The use of complementary and alternative medications for metabolic syndrome has limited literature support. Traditional Chinese medicines may have a role, as a variety of agents, including ginseng, berberine, and bitter gourd, have demonstrated some favorable metabolic effects, but large-scale clinical trials are needed to fully investigate their safety and efficacy.[19]

A variety of other complementary and alternative treatments may have a potential role in the management of metabolic syndrome[20] and additional study remains warranted.

Diet

Lifestyle change and weight loss are considered the most important initial steps in treating metabolic syndrome. Studies comparing ethnically similar populations exposed to different dietary environments suggested that Westernized diets are strongly associated with a higher risk of developing metabolic syndrome.[4]

On the other hand, diets rich in dairy, fish, and cereal grains may be associated with a lower risk of developing metabolic syndrome.[21,22] Not surprisingly, Mediterranean-style diets appear to be associated with a much lower risk and possibly with resolution of metabolic syndrome in patients who have met diagnostic criteria, especially when coupled with adequate exercise regimens.[23]

Bangladeshi diet such as fish, rice, vegetable, and daal are having less calorie. A meta-analysis of multiple population studies associated chocolate consumption with a substantial risk reduction (approximately 30%) for cardiometabolic disorders, including coronary disease, cardiac deaths, diabetes, and stroke.[24]

Activity

Exercise is thought to be an important intervention,[25] and the current recommendation is for patients to perform regular moderate-intensity physical activity for at least 30 minutes continuously at least 5 days per week (ideally, 7 days per week). Maintaining long-term adherence, however, remains a challenge.[26] Achieving moderate intensity activity for 120–150 minutes a week may reduce the risk of developing metabolic syndrome.[27] Among patients who already have metabolic syndrome, physical activity correlates with a much lower (about 50%) risk of developing coronary heart disease.[28]

Evidence suggests that excessive sitting and other behaviors that are low in activity and energy expenditure may trigger unique cellular responses that contribute to the development of metabolic syndrome.[29]

Obviously, such a course of action could prove to be inadequate and additional pharmacological treatment of insulin resistance, obesity, dyslipidemia, or hypertension could be required.[30]

DETERRENCE AND PREVENTION

Hypertension

Regular blood pressure screening, lifestyle modification, and drug therapy are recommended. A lower risk of stroke and cardiovascular events are seen when systolic blood pressure levels are <140 mm Hg and diastolic blood pressure is <90 mm Hg. In patients who have hypertension with diabetes or renal disease, the blood pressure goal is <130/80 mm Hg.

Diabetes

Blood pressure control is recommended in type 1 and 2 diabetes. Hypertensive agents that are useful in the diabetic population include angiotensin-converting enzyme (ACE) inhibitors or angiotensin receptor blockers (ARBs).

Treating adults with diabetes with statin therapy, especially patients with other risk factors, is recommended, and monotherapy with fibrates may also be considered to lower stroke risk. Taking aspirin is reasonable in patients who are at high CVD risk. However, the benefit of taking aspirin in diabetic patients for the reduction of stroke risk has not been fully demonstrated.

Dyslipidemia

Statin therapy is recommended in patients with coronary heart disease and certain high-risk conditions for the primary prevention of ischemic stroke. In addition to statin therapy, therapeutic lifestyle changes are also recommended.

Diet and Nutrition

Metabolic syndrome is basically a lifestyle disease. It is a constellation of metabolic abnormalities that confer an increased risk of CVD and diabetes mellitus.

Diet with less refined carbohydrate, polysaturated fat, and low salt is recommended. Diets that promote the consumption of fruits, vegetables, and low-fat dairy products, such as the DASH (Dietary Approaches to Stop Hypertension)—style diet, help to lower blood pressure and may lower the risk of stroke. "Healthy" diet, for example, <5 g of salt per day (British Hypertension Society guidelines), <300 mg of cholesterol per day, 1–1.2 g of calcium, and 800 IU of vitamin D3 per day, which could be achieved, inter alia, by reducing fat intake (including saturated fats) and carbohydrates intake (including sugars), increased consumption of fruit, vegetables, and marine fish.

Giving up smoking, alcohol, and intellectual activity may help to prevent metabolic syndrome.

■ PHYSICAL ACTIVITY

Increases in physical activity are associated with a reduction in the risk of stroke. The goal is to engage in at least 30 minutes of moderate intensity activity on a daily basis.

Obesity and Body Fat Distribution

Weight reduction among persons who are overweight or obese is recommended to reduce blood pressure and risk of stroke.

Sleep Health

Care should be taken to ensure that patients with metabolic syndrome practice healthy sleep behaviors, even in patients who do not have sleep apnea or suspected sleep apnea, some studies have suggested a relationship between sleep deprivation or inadequate sleep time and metabolic syndrome.[31] Shift workers, who tend to have poor quality sleep, may also be at higher risk of developing metabolic syndrome.[32]

■ MEDICATION SUMMARY

An insulin-sensitizing agent, such as metformin, is typically used at the start of hyperglycemia treatment in patients with metabolic syndrome. Some literature suggests that metformin may help to reverse the pathophysiologic changes of metabolic syndrome. This includes when it is used in combination with lifestyle changes[33] or with peroxisome proliferator-activated receptor agonists, such as fibrates[34] and thiazolidinediones (e.g., pioglitazone, rosiglitazone),[35,36] each of which may produce favorable metabolic alterations as single agents in patients with metabolic syndrome.[37]

Aspirin may contribute to the primary prevention of cardiovascular complications in metabolic syndrome, particularly in patients with at least an intermediate risk of suffering a cardiovascular event (i.e., >6%, 10-year risk).[38,39]

Additional therapies have found early support from more recent data. For example, a small trial of high-dose resveratrol therapy (1,000 mg daily) was found to lead to greater new bone formation and mineralization with metabolic syndrome:[40,41]
- Lipid-lowering agents
- Statins
- Antihyertensive
- Antiplatelets.

Aspirin is a stronger inhibitor of prostaglandin synthesis and platelet aggregation than are other salicylic acid derivatives.

Aspirin irreversibly inhibits platelet aggregation by inhibiting platelet cyclooxygenase. This, in turn, inhibits conversion of arachidonic acid to prostaglandin I2 (potent vasodilator and inhibitor of platelet activation) and thromboxane A2 (potent vasoconstrictor and platelet aggregating agent). Platelet inhibition lasts for the life of the cell (approximately 10 days).

Aspirin may be used in low dose to inhibit platelet aggregation and improve complications of venous stasis and thrombosis. It reduces the likelihood of myocardial infarction and is also very effective in reducing the risk of stroke.

According to the current data, hormone therapy (HT) is not recommended as a prevention strategy for metabolic disorders in menopause. However, as part of a comprehensive strategy to prevent chronic disease after menopause, menopausal HT, particularly estrogen therapy (ET) may be considered as part of the armamentarium.[42] The choice of a specific therapy should always be aligned with a particular patient and adapted to her condition and health needs, which might require consultation and further management by a range of medical professionals.

KEY MESSAGES

- Metabolic syndrome is defined as assemblage of risk factors for CVD, the emergence of which is at high point in postmenopausal women.
- The diagnosis of metabolic syndrome helps to identify menopausal patients at increased long-term risk for cardiovascular diseases, type 2 diabetes mellitus and ischemic stroke.
- Metabolic disorders occurring in menopause, including dyslipidemia, disorders of carbohydrate metabolism (IGT, T2DM), or components of metabolic syndrome, constitute risk factors for CVD in women.
- Undiagnosed and untreated, metabolic disorders may adversely affect the health and quality of women's life. Prevention and treatment preceded by early diagnosis should be the main goal for the physicians involved in menopausal care.
- Hormone therapy is not recommend as a preventive strategy for metabolic disorders in menopause. Nevertheless, as part of a comprehensive strategy to prevent chronic diseases after menopause, menopausal hormonal therapy and particularly estrogen therapy (ET) may be considered (after balancing benefits/risks and excluding women with absolute contraindications to this therapy).
- Lifestyle modifications, with moderate physical activity and healthy diet at the forefront, should be still the first choice recommendation for all women of menopause as this is the window opportunity. By adopting this strategy women may enjoy healthy aging.

REFERENCES

1. Olufadi R, Byrne CD. Clinical and laboratory diagnosis of the metabolic syndrome. J Clin Pathol. 2008;61(6):697-706.
2. Hernandez-Baixauli J, Quesada-Vázquez S, Mariné-Casadó R, Gil Cardoso K, Caimari A, Del Bas JM, et al. Detection of early disease risk factors associated with metabolic syndrome: a new era with the NMR metabolomics assessment. Nutrients. 2020;12(3):806.
3. Ben Ali S, Belfki-Benali H, Aounallah-Skhiri H, Traissac P, Maire B, Delpeuch F, et al. Menopause and metabolic syndrome in tunisian women. Biomed Res Int. 2014;2014:457131.

4. Yoneda M, Yamane K, Jitsuiki K, Nakanishi S, Kamei N, Watanabe H, et al. Prevalence of metabolic syndrome compared between native Japanese and Japanese-Americans. Diabetes Res Clin Pract. 2008;79(3):518-22.
5. Toth MJ, Sites CK, Poehlman ET, Tchernof A. Effect of menopausal status on lipolysis: comparison of plasma glycerol levels in middle-aged, premenopausal and early, postmenopausal women. Metabolism. 2002;51:322-6.
6. Bagnoli VR, Fonseca AM, Arie WM, Das Neves EM, Azevedo RS, Sorpreso IC, et al. Metabolic disorder and obesity in 5027 Brazilian postmenopausal women. Gynecol Endocrinol. 2014;30:717-20.
7. Waki H, Tontonoz P. Endocrine functions of adipose tissue. Annu Rev Pathol. 2007;2:31-56.
8. Reaven G, Abbasi F, McLaughlin T. Obesity, insulin resistance, and cardiovascular disease. Recent Prog Horm Res. 2004;59:207-23.
9. Matsuzawa Y. Therapy insight: adipocytokines in metabolic syndrome and related cardiovascular disease. Nat Clin Pract Cardiovasc Med. 2006;3:35-42.
10. Heima NE, Eekhoff EM, Oosterwerff MM, Lips PT, van Schoor NM, Simsek S. Thyroid function and the metabolic syndrome in older persons: a population-based study. Eur J Endocrinol. 2013;168:59-65.
11. Puig JG, Martinez MA. Hyperuricemia, gout and the metabolic syndrome. Curr Opin Rheumatol. 2008;20:187-91.
12. Welty FK, Alfaddagh A, Elajami TK. Targeting inflammation in metabolic syndrome. Transl Res. 2016;167:257-80.
13. Tupper T, Gopalakrishnan G. Prevention of diabetes development in those with the metabolic syndrome. Med Clin North Am. 2007;91:1091-105, viii-ix.
14. James PA, Oparil S, Carter BL, Cushman WC, Dennison-Himmelfarb C, Handler J, et al. 2014 evidence-based guideline for the management of high blood pressure in adults: report from the panel members appointed to the Eighth Joint National Committee (JNC 8). JAMA. 2014;311:507-20.
15. Eckel RH, Jakicic JM, Ard JD, de Jesus JM, Houston Miller N, Hubbard VS, et al. 2013 AHA/ACC guideline on lifestyle management to reduce cardiovascular risk: a report of the American College of Cardiology/American Heart Association Task Force on Practice Guidelines. J Am Coll Cardiol. 2014;63(25 Pt B):2960-84.
16. Jensen MD, Ryan DH, Apovian CM, Ard JD, Comuzzie AG, Donato KA, et al. 2013 AHA/ACC/TOS guideline for the management of overweight and obesity in adults: a report of the American College of Cardiology/American Heart Association Task Force on Practice Guidelines and The Obesity Society. J Am Coll Cardiol. 2014;63(25 Pt B):2985-3023.
17. Kini S, Herron DM, Yanagisawa RT. Bariatric surgery for morbid obesity—a cure for metabolic syndrome? Med Clin North Am. 2007;91:1255-71, xi.
18. Bagry HS, Raghavendran S, Carli F. Metabolic syndrome and insulin resistance: perioperative considerations. Anesthesiology. 2008;108:506-23.
19. Yin J, Zhang H, Ye J. Traditional Chinese medicine in treatment of metabolic syndrome. Endocr Metab Immune Disord Drug Targets. 2008;8:99-111.
20. Hollander JM, Mechanick JI. Complementary and alternative medicine and the management of the metabolic syndrome. J Am Diet Assoc. 2008;108:495-509.
21. Ruidavets JB, Bongard V, Dallongeville J, Arveiler D, Ducimetière P, Perret B, et al. High consumptions of grain, fish, dairy products and combinations of these are associated with a low prevalence of metabolic syndrome. J Epidemiol Community Health. 2007;61:810-7.
22. Mattei J, Bhupathiraju S, Tucker KL. Higher adherence to a diet score based on American Heart Association recommendations is associated with lower odds of allostatic load and metabolic syndrome in Puerto Rican adults. J Nutr. 2013;143:1753-9.
23. Esposito K, Ciotola M, Giugliano D. Mediterranean diet and the metabolic syndrome. Mol Nutr Food Res. 2007;51:1268-74.

24. Buitrago-Lopez A, Sanderson J, Johnson L, Warnakula S, Wood A, Di Angelantonio E, et al. Chocolate consumption and cardiometabolic disorders: systematic review and meta-analysis. BMJ. 2011;343:d4488.
25. Roberts CK, Hevener AL, Barnard RJ. Metabolic syndrome and insulin resistance: underlying causes and modification by exercise training. Compr Physiol. 2013;3: 1-58.
26. Fappa E, Yannakoulia M, Pitsavos C, Skoumas I, Valourdou S, Stefanadis C. Lifestyle intervention in the management of metabolic syndrome: could we improve adherence issues? Nutrition. 2008;24:286-91.
27. Department of Health and Human Services, Centers for Disease Control and Prevention. (2021). Physical activity: Benefits of physical activity. [online] Available from http://www.cdc.gov/physicalactivity/basics/pa-health/index.htm [Last accessed March, 2021].
28. Broekhuizen LN, Boekholdt SM, Arsenault BJ, Despres JP, Stroes ES, Kastelein JJ, et al. Physical activity, metabolic syndrome, and coronary risk: the EPIC-Norfolk prospective population study. Eur J Cardiovasc Prev Rehabil. 2011;18:209-17.
29. Hamilton MT, Hamilton DG, Zderic TW. Role of low energy expenditure and sitting in obesity, metabolic syndrome, type 2 diabetes, and cardiovascular disease. Diabetes. 2007;56:2655-67.
30. The Writing Group on behalf of the Workshop Consensus Group. Aging, menopause, cardiovascular disease and HRT. International Menopause Society Consensus Statement. Climacteric. 2009;12:368-77.
31. Hall MH, Muldoon MF, Jennings JR, Buysse DJ, Flory JD, Manuck SB. Self-reported sleep duration is associated with the metabolic syndrome in midlife adults. Sleep. 2008;31:635-43.
32. Kawada T, Otsuka T. Effect of shift work on the development of metabolic syndrome after 3 years in Japanese male workers. Arch Environ Occup Health. 2014;69:55-61.
33. Orchard TJ, Temprosa M, Goldberg R, Haffner S, Ratner R, Marcovina S, et al. The effect of metformin and intensive lifestyle intervention on the metabolic syndrome: the Diabetes Prevention Program randomized trial. Ann Intern Med. 2005;142: 611-9.
34. Nieuwdorp M, Stroes ES, Kastelein JJ. Normalization of metabolic syndrome using fenofibrate, metformin or their combination. Diabetes Obes Metab. 2007;9:869-78.
35. Derosa G, D'Angelo A, Ragonesi PD, Ciccarelli L, Piccinni MN, Pricolo F, et al. Metabolic effects of pioglitazone and rosiglitazone in patients with diabetes and metabolic syndrome treated with metformin. Intern Med J. 2007;37:79-86.
36. Di Pino A, DeFronzo RA. Insulin resistance and atherosclerosis: implications for insulin-sensitizing agents. Endocr Rev. 2019;40:1447-67.
37. Bragt MC, Popeijus HE. Peroxisome proliferator-activated receptors and the metabolic syndrome. Physiol Behav. 2008;94:187-97.
38. Shields TM, Hennekens CH. Management of metabolic syndrome: aspirin. Endocrinol Metab Clin North Am. 2004;33:577-93, vii.
39. Blaha MJ, Bansal S, Rouf R, Golden SH, Blumenthal RS, Defilippis AP. A practical "ABCDE" approach to the metabolic syndrome. Mayo Clin Proc. 2008;83:932-41.
40. McCall B. (2014). Medscape Medical News: Resveratrol boosts bone formation in obese men. [online] Available from http://www.medscape.com/viewarticle/833807 [Last accessed January, 2021].
41. Ornstrup MJ, Harslof T, Kjaer TN, Langdahl BL, Pedersen SB. Resveratrol increases bone mineral density and bone alkaline phosphatase in obese men: a randomized placebo-controlled trial. J Clin Endocrinol Metab. 2014;99:4720-9.
42. Stachowiak G, Zając A, Pertyński T. Zespół metaboliczny u kobiet w okresie menopauzy. Prz Menopauzalny. 2009;8:6-10.

Postmenopausal Bleeding

CHAPTER

▪ INTRODUCTION

Postmenopausal bleeding (PMB) is considered at least 12 months after the last normal period. The incidence of PMB appears to correlate with the time since menopause. Unscheduled bleeding is defined as noncyclical bleeding in menopause women taking hormone replacement therapy. Although PMB usually has benign causes, the priority is to exclude malignancy.

Postmenopausal bleeding is a common clinical problem accounts approximately 5% of gynecology office visits.[1]

All postmenopausal women with unexpected vaginal bleeding should be evaluated for endometrial carcinoma since this potentially lethal disease will be the cause of bleeding in approximately 10% range (1-25%), depending upon risk factors.[2] For PMB endometrial carcinoma must be regarded until proven otherwise. Management of PMB is aimed at excluding cervical carcinoma, endometrial carcinoma precancerous endometrial changes and then to treat the real cause. A negative test guarantees the normality; but the clinician should be aware of the possibility of a false negative result. PMB usually attributed to an intrauterine source, but may arise from the cervix, vagina, vulva, fallopian tubes, or be related to ovarian pathology (hormone producing tumor).

The origin of bleeding can also involve non-gynecologic sites, such as the urethra, bladder, anus/rectum/bowel, or perineum. In postmenopausal women cervical stenosis may occur which inhibit egress of blood from the uterine cavity; therefore hematometra may result.

The differential diagnosis of bleeding in postmenopausal women is less broad than that for abnormal uterine bleeding in premenopausal women since the various causes of anovulation are not relevant here.

▪ DIFFERENTIAL DIAGNOSIS OF POSTMENOPAUSAL BLEEDING

- Vaginal atrophy—the most common cause of PMB
- Indiscriminate use of menopause hormone therapy (MHT), tamoxifen
- Endometrial hyperplasia (EH) with atypia and without atypia
- Endometrial cancer
- Endometrial polyps or infection
- Cervical cancer; need to check if the cervical smear is up to date. Cervical polyp
- Cervical ulcer caused by uterine prolapse
- Uterine sarcoma (rare)

- Ovarian cancer, especially estrogen-secreting (theca cell) ovarian tumors
- Vaginal cancer (very uncommon)
- Vulvar cancer may bleed, but the lesion should be obvious
- Nongynecological causes including trauma or a bleeding disorder.

Other causes: Lesions and cracks of the vulva, trauma, phytoestrogens, and forgotten pessaries.

Though benign conditions are the most common causes of PMB, but it needs to be considered seriously by the patients and clinicians, as it may be the first warning symptoms of an underlying malignancy, which if diagnosed early can be cured completely.

Association of PMB

Atrophy: Hypoestrogenism causes atrophy of the endometrium and vagina. In the uterus, the collapsed, atrophic endometrial surfaces contain little or no fluid to prevent intracavitary friction.[3] This results in microerosions of the surface epithelium and a subsequent chronic inflammatory reaction (chronic endometritis), which is prone to light bleeding or spotting.

Classic vaginal findings of atrophy include a pale, dry vaginal epithelium that is smooth and shiny with loss of most rugae. If inflammation is present, additional findings may include patchy erythema, petechiae, blood vessels visible through the thinned out epithelium, friability, bleeding, and discharge.

Cancer: Approximately 6-19% of women with postmenopausal vaginal bleeding have endometrial cancer.[4,5] Different studies showed that risk of endometrial cancer in the setting of PMB increases with increasing age after menopause.[6] Age > 55 years, history of recurrent bleeding episodes, and bleeding volume exceeding five pads per day were significantly associated with endometrial cancer.

■ RISK FACTORS FOR ENDOMETRIAL CANCER

- Chronic estrogen activities/chronic anovulation
- Unopposed estrogen-only therapy
- *Tamoxifen use*: It has an antiestrogen effect on the breast, but a proestrogen effect on the uterus and bones
- Obesity
- Early menarche and late menopause
- Increasing age
- Estrogen secreting tumor
- Hereditary nonpolyposis colorectal carcinoma
- Lynch syndrome
- *Potential heritable factors*: Cowden syndrome, multiple hamartoma syndrome
- BRCA carriers
- *Uncertain factors*: Diabetes, hypertension, phytoestrogens.[7]

In a meta-analysis of observational studies, the pooled prevalence of PMB among patients with endometrial cancer was 91% (95% CI 87–93), irrespective of tumor stage.[8] Pelvic examination is usually normal in patients with early-stage disease. In more advanced disease, the uterus may be enlarged and/or fixed in the pelvis. In postmenopausal patients, uterine imaging may show a thickened endometrium and endometrial biopsy reveals diagnosis.

Polyps: Polyps are benign endometrial growths of unknown etiology that are a common cause of perimenopausal and early postmenopausal uterine bleeding. Growth of polyps can be stimulated by estrogen therapy or tamoxifen. The definite etiology of endometrial polyps is unknown. However, endometrial polyps are associated with EH; therefore, unopposed estrogen is considered to be a risk factor.[9] The prevalence of malignant endometrial polyps in the symptomatic postmenopausal female is 4.47% compared with 1.51% in an asymptomatic postmenopausal female.[10] Additional risk factors for malignant endometrial polyps include age greater than 60, large-sized polyps, menopause status, symptomatic bleeding, and polycystic ovarian syndrome.[11] Chronic tamoxifen use has been associated with the development of EH, polyps and endometrial cancer. Transvaginal ultrasound (TVS) shows increased endometrial thickness (ET) greater than 4 mm is related to endometrial pathology, including polyps.[12] The location of the polyp, number, and diameter does not correlate with the reported symptoms.[13]

Saline infusion sonography (SIS) or hysteroscopy are good alternative. Hysteroscopic polypectomy with endometrial biopsy is gold standard. Blind tissue sampling with endometrial biopsy or dilation and curettage (D&C) procedure is inaccurate in the diagnosis of endometrial polyps and should only be used in settings where hysteroscopic treatment is unavailable.[14] Histopathology showing polyp with atypia or recurrence of polyp carries potential for malignancy. Hysterectomy should be the preferred treatment in this case.

Endometrial hyperplasia: One of the important causes of PMB is EH. Since postmenopausal women should be estrogen deficient, EH at this time it is abnormal and requires a usual explanation. Low dose estrogen and microvascular changes of endometrium by progesterone are associated with bleeding. MHT may cause spotting for couple of weeks but it usually improves by 6 months of time. Endogenous estrogen production from ovarian or adrenal tumors is also the possible causes of hyperplasia. Obese women also have high levels of endogenous estrogen due to the conversion of androstenedione to estrone and the aromatization of androgens to estradiol, both of which occur in peripheral adipose tissue. Also, EH frequently results from chronic estrogen stimulation unopposed by the counterbalancing effects of progesterone.[15]

The presence of nuclear atypia is the most important indicator of the risk of endometrial carcinoma. It is sometimes difficult to distinguish a precursor lesion from endometrial carcinoma. EH is also known as endometrial intraepithelial neoplasia (EIN).

Endometrial hyperplasia/intraepithelial neoplasia typically presents with abnormal uterine bleeding in postmenopausal women. EH/intraepithelial neoplasm is a histologic diagnosis made with sampling of the endometrium. Neither endometrial biopsy nor D&C procedure detect all cases of endometrial carcinoma; up to 10% are falsely negative.

Leiomyomata uteri: Leiomyomata uteri (fibroids) are the most common pelvic tumors in women. The prevalence in postmenopausal women is one-tenth that of premenopausal women, thus they are a potential, but uncommon, cause of uterine bleeding in menopausal women.[16] The diagnosis of a uterine sarcoma should be considered in postmenopausal women with presumed uterine leiomyomas producing symptoms.

Sarcomas of the uterus constitute only 3-5% of all uterine tumors and may present with PMB. These cancers arise from the stroma of the endometrium (endometrial stromal sarcomas) or the myometrium. They may look and feel like benign leiomyomas. Endometrial histology may be normal; diagnosis requires a hysterectomy.

Fallopian tube or ovarian cancer can cause postmenopausal uterine bleeding. Cervical and vaginal cancers typically present with vaginal bleeding. Vulvar cancers are not associated with bleeding until they are advanced.

Choriocarcinoma is a rare cause of uterine bleeding in menopausal women.

Postradiation therapy: Vaginal bleeding can be a late effect of radiation therapy.[17]

Anticoagulant therapy: Use of anticoagulants may rarely cause uterine bleeding.

Herbal and dietary supplements: Soy and other phytoestrogens in large doses may be associated with EH.[18]

Infection: Endometritis is an uncommon cause of PMB. In the developing world, however, endometrial tuberculosis may present as PMB.[19-21]

Postmenopausal hormone therapy: Many postmenopausal women who take estrogen therapy develop vaginal bleeding; the frequency depends upon the regimen and the doses used. Usually within 6 months' time, it gets well.

Diseases of the urethra (e.g., urethritis), bladder (e.g., cancer or urinary tract infection), and bowel (e.g., inflammatory bowel disease or hemorrhoids) may cause bleeding that is mistaken for genital tract bleeding. These disorders should be considered and evaluated for in patients with bleeding in whom there is no obvious genital tract etiology. A radiograph of the pelvis to rule out fracture should be considered when there is genital bleeding after trauma, in a postmenopausal woman with osteoporosis.

EVALUATION

Primary evaluation of women with PMB should include detailed medical history, clinical examination, and TVS with evaluation of ET, with or without endometrial smpling.[4] According to the American College of Obstetricians and Gynecologists (ACOG), the clinical approach to PMB requires prompt and efficient evaluation to exclude or diagnose carcinoma. Women with PMB may be assessed initially with either endometrial biopsy or TVS. This initial evaluation does not require performance of both tests. TVS can be useful in the triage of patients in whom endometrial sampling was performed but tissue was insufficient for diagnosis. When TVS is performed for patients with PMB and an ET of less than or equal to 4 mm is found, endometrial sampling is not required. Meaningful assessment of the endometrium by ultrasonography is not possible in all patients. In such cases, alternative assessment should be completed. When bleeding persists despite negative initial evaluations, additional assessment usually is indicated.[22]

Endometrial cancer can reasonably be excluded by ultrasound in postmenopausal women with a thin (≤4 mm), homogeneous endometrium. Endometrial biopsy is required if:
- If repeated bleeding episodes for women who showed normal findings on primary evaluation
- The endometrial lining is thicker than 4 mm
- The endometrium shows diffuse or focal increased echogenicity (heterogeneity)
- The endometrium is not adequately visualized on sonography
- The woman has persistent bleeding.

The risk of endometrial cancer is low when the ET is less than 4 mm.[23-26] With nonrepresentative/uncertain findings on endometrial biopsy, the cause of bleeding can be atrophic endometrial lining, however, malignancy should be excluded. Differential diagnosis of bleeding from the urinary tract or bowel should be excluded.

History

A detailed history on duration, frequency, length and quantity of bleeding and its relationship to coitus, pain should be established. Menstrual history, parity, past medical history and family history are important in evaluation of PMB. Any risk factors need to be elicited. Is there a family history of breast, colon, and endometrial cancer? What is the medical history and are any medications being taken (e.g., hormones therapy, anticoagulants)?

Women with a family history of hereditary nonpolyposis colorectal cancer have a lifetime risk of developing endometrial cancer of around 42-60%. They usually develop cancer before menopause. History of liver diseases needs to be focused.

Evaluation needs general examination and thorough physical examination of the external and internal anatomy of the female genital tract. The focus of the evaluation is to determine the bleeding site; to note any suspicious lesions, lacerations, or foreign bodies; and to assess the size, contour, and tenderness of the uterus. Lower genital tract (vulva, vagina, ectocervix) causes of bleeding can usually be excluded by a normal physical examination.

Clinical Examination
- Speculum examination
- Bi manual vaginal examination
- Digital rectal examination (DRE).

Investigation
Transvaginal ultrasound is used to measure ET is the mainstay to evaluate endometrium. Color Doppler is good adjustment to ET, if ET is <4 m then may not require any further investigation unless there is persistent or recurrence of bleeding. If ET is >4 mm endometrial biopsy must be performed. Clinical judgment should be used when there is recurrent PMB.

Definite diagnosis of PMB is made by histopathology by endometrial sampling or D&C procedure. *Hysteroscopy (gold standard for evaluation)* adjunct investigations are done to exclude other different diseases.

Transvaginal ultrasound is appropriate for initial evaluation of PMB. If the endometrium has a thickness >4 mm, further evaluation is necessary. If bleeding persists or recurs, endometrial sampling is indicated. TVS, SIS, repeated endometrial biopsy, diagnostic hysteroscopy with endometrial biopsy can be done. Hysteroscopic evaluation and guided biopsy is the gold standard. Diagnostic hysteroscopy provides direct visualization of the endometrial cavity, thereby allowing targeted biopsy or excision of lesions identified during the procedure. A D&C alone (approximately 60% of curettage specimens sample less than half of the uterine cavity so there is chance of missing pathology).[27]

Obesity, uterine position, or myometrium abnormalities may preclude satisfactory endometrial assessment with TVS. In these cases, PMB should be evaluated with sonohysterography, office hysteroscopy, or endometrial sampling. If such sampling yields insufficient tissue for diagnosis, further evaluation might not be necessary, provided subsequent TVS demonstrates an ET ≤ 4 mm and bleeding does not recur. When postmenopausal women without bleeding undergo TVS for indications such as pelvic pain or adnexal pathology, an ET >4 mm may be incidentally found, additional endometrial assessment is not routinely indicated. Endometrial cancer can reasonably be excluded by ultrasound in postmenopausal women with a ET ≤ 4 mm.

Persistent bleeding can be a sign of endometrial cancer even when the ET is less than 4–5 mm since a thin or indistinct endometrial stripe does not reliably exclude type 2 endometrial cancer.[28,29] Therefore, women with persistent bleeding should be evaluated further.

Cervical cytology: The mean age of cervical cancer diagnosis is 52.2 years; the distribution of cases is bimodal, with peaks at 35–39 years and 60–64 years.[30] All women need cervical cancer screening as a part of the evaluation of abnormal bleeding, as it can be difficult to distinguish between endocervical and upper uterine bleeding. Using ThinPrep, the same specimen can be used for analysis of both cytology and human papillomavirus.

Any visible lesion needs to be biopsied, even if the cytology is normal.[31]

Saline infusion sonography, magnetic resonance imaging (MRI), and computed tomography (CT) scans are reserved for special cases.

■ TREATMENT

In postmenopausal women, uterine bleeding is usually light and self-limited. Treatment is focused toward the cause. But exclusion of cancer is the main objective. However, treatment is otherwise dependent on findings during the diagnostic evaluation.

Regarding management of EH it is determined by clinical factors and by histological classification. The three most common options for the management of EH are surveillance, progestin therapy, and hysterectomy.

Clinical factors need to be considered are—obesity, ovulatory dysfunction, increased genetic risk, and increased age. Although, EH and endometrial cancer can be observed in younger women commonly in those with polycystic ovary syndrome and body mass index >30 kg/m^2.[32]

The ET on TVS ≥20 mm has a greater risk for concomitant endometrial cancer.[33,34]

We need to follow 2014 World Health Organization classification criteria, i.e.:
- Hyperplasia without atypia
- Hyperplasia with atypia.[35]

For *postmenopausal women* with EH without atypia, repeat endometrial biopsy is performed every 3–6 months for up to 1 year until the biopsy shows normal endometrium. They may be treated with the levonorgestrel-releasing intrauterine system (LNG-IUS) and have rates of regression to normal endometrium of approximately 90%. A systematic review of 24 observational studies including 1,001 participants found that treatment with LNG 52 compared with oral progestins had a higher regression rate for complex EH (92 vs. 66%).[36] Patients with EH without atypia treated with the LNG 52 have rates of regression to normal endometrium of approximately 90%.[37]

Hysterectomy is advised if normal endometrium is not achieved, if atypical EH or endometrial carcinoma develops, or if no improvement.

Postmenopausal women having EH with atypia EIN needs special counseling, as malignant potential is very high. Coexistent endometrial carcinoma may be present at hysterectomy in approximately 37% of women with a preoperative diagnosis of atypical EH.[38] The risk of progression of atypical EH to endometrial carcinoma is 15–28%, based on studies with up to 20 years of follow-up.[39]

Hysterectomy is the choice of option, though progestin therapy with LNG-IUS (52 mg) with a release rate of 20 μg/day over 5 years, has been shown regression of atypical EH and grade 1 endometrial carcinoma in up to 75–85% of women.[40] However, hysterectomy is curative and thus is still the preferred treatment.

Maintenance Therapy

For women with EH on progestin therapy, after regression to normal endometrium, maintenance progestin therapy may be required indefinitely if patients have risk factors for endometrial carcinoma (e.g., obesity, diabetes, polycystic ovary syndrome). Some women may have persistent or recurrent abnormal uterine bleeding, despite no disease progression on serial endometrial sampling. In such cases, hysterectomy may be offered.

Risk of relapse: A cohort study with long-term follow-up showed a relapse rate of 12.7% for hyperplasia without atypia.[41]

A review of patients with atypical EH managed with progestin therapy showed a recurrence rate of 23.2%.[40]

For patients who have a relapse of EH, consideration is given to either continuous progestin therapy or to hysterectomy.

Specific Treatment in PMB

Atrophic vaginitis: Local estrogen treatment is given in women suffering from vaginal atrophy.[42]

Endometrial polyps: Hysteroscopy is gold standard to visualize endometrium thoroughly. Polypectomy and the histopathological examination is the treatment. Simultaneous endometrium sampling for histopathology is necessary as the possibility of hyperplasia is high (e.g., 3% of endometrial polyps). If hysteroscopy is not available. Dilatation polypectomy and endometrial curettage can be done.

Other polyps: Cervical polypectomy is the treatment for cervical polyp. But endometrial curettage should be done to exclude any endometrial pathology.

Endometrial thickness <4 mm: Follow-up with a repeat ultrasonography need to be done unless continuous bleeding occurs.

Endometrial thickness >4 mm: Endometrial sampling with hysteroscopy. EH without atypia responds well to cyclic progestin treatment. After 3 months a repeat endometrial biopsy may be considered to confirm absence of hyperplasia. Levonorgestrel intrauterine system is preferred over systemic treatment. Refractory patients may need hysterectomy.

Hyperplasia with atypia: Definitive treatment for postmenopausal women is surgery, medical treatment only after in-depth counseling.

Endometrial carcinoma and cervical carcinoma: They may need surgery and/or chemotherapy or radiation therapy according to the protocol.

Endometrial Safety, Bleeding and Menopausal Hormonal Therapy

Adequate endometrial protection was demonstrated in MHT users with sequential and continuous micronized progesterone (MPA). The LNG-IUS with estrogen has been reported to be more effective than sequential MPA/other progestins for endometrial protection.

More recently, a regimen combining the selective estrogen receptor modulator, bazedoxifene, with conjugated equine estrogens has been introduced as a progestogen-free alternative for MHT in women with a uterus. Tibolone is also used extensively as a form of MHT. It should not be used before 1 year of menopause as during this period irregular bleeding may occur.

■ KEY MESSAGES

- Postmenopausal bleeding is "endometrial cancer until proven otherwise", although only 1–14% of such patients will actually have cancer.
- Prompt evaluation is essential to find out the genital, nongynecological and others sources. Risk factors for endometrial cancer need to be assessed for each case.
- Initial evaluation is by TVS, if ET is <4 mm no further evaluation is required but follow-up consultation must be taken. If ET is >4 mm, hysteroscopy evaluation and endometrial sampling is recommended (Gold Standard).
- Blind endometrial sampling is not accurate as it only reveals when endometrial cancer exceeds more than 50% of the endometrial surface area so may be done if hysteroscopy evaluation is not possible.
- Higher doses of progesterone may be required for endometrial protection when higher doses of estradiol are used, for hormone therapy or in women with high body mass index.
- Unopposed estrogen therapy should not be used if women have uterus as it is associated with a duration and dose-related increase in risk of EH and cancer.
- Endometrial protection requires an adequate dose and duration of progestogen.
- Finally, patient counseling and shared decision is the cornerstone of success to address PMB.

REFERENCES

1. Moodley M, Roberts C. Clinical pathway for the evaluation of postmenopausal bleeding with an emphasis on endometrial cancer detection. J Obstet Gynaecol. 2004;24:736.
2. Prendergast EN, Misch E, Chou YA, Roston A, Patel A. Insufficient endometrial biopsy results in women with abnormal uterine bleeding. Obstet Gynecol. 2014;123(Suppl 1):180S.
3. Ferenczy A. Pathophysiology of endometrial bleeding. Maturitas. 2003;45:1.
4. Van Hanegem N, Breijer MC, Khan KS, Clark TJ, Burger MP, Mol BM, et al. Diagnostic evaluation of the endometrium in postmenopausal bleeding: an evidence-based approach. Maturitas. 2011;68:155-64.
5. Cote ML, Ruterbusch JJ, Ahmed Q, Bandyopadhyay S, Alosh B, Abdulfatah E, et al. Endometrial cancer in morbidly obese women: do racial disparities affect surgical or survival outcomes? Gynecol Oncol. 2014;133:38.
6. Salman MC, Bozdag G, Dogan S, Yuce K. Role of postmenopausal bleeding pattern and women's age in the prediction of endometrial cancer. Aust N Z J Obstet Gynaecol. 2013;53:484.
7. Lee-may C, Berek JS. Endometrial carcinoma: epidemiology, risk factors, and prevention: UpTodate. 2020.
8. Clarke MA, Long BJ, Del Mar Morillo A, Arbyn M, Bakkum-Gamez JN, Wentzensen N. Association of endometrial cancer risk with postmenopausal bleeding in women: a systematic review and meta-analysis. JAMA Intern Med. 2018;178:1210.
9. Tanos V, Berry KE, Seikkula J, Abi Raad E, Stavroulis A, Sleiman Z, et al. The management of polyps in female reproductive organs. Int J Surg. 2017;43:7-16.
10. Lee SC, Kaunitz AM, Sanchez-Ramos L, Rhatigan RM. The oncogenic potential of endometrial polyps: a systematic review and meta-analysis. Obstet Gynecol. 2010;116(5):1197-205.
11. Elfayomy AK, Soliman BS. Risk Factors Associated with the Malignant Changes of Symptomatic and Asymptomatic Endometrial Polyps in Premenopausal Women. J Obstet Gynaecol India. 2015;65(3):186-92.
12. Maia H, Barbosa IC, Marques D, Calmon LC, Ladipo OA, Coutinho EM. Hysteroscopy and transvaginal sonography in menopausal women receiving hormone replacement therapy. J Am Assoc Gynecol Laparosc. 1996;4(1):13-8.
13. Hassa H, Tekin B, Senses T, Kaya M, Karatas A. Are the site, diameter, and number of endometrial polyps related with symptomatology? Am J Obstet. Gynecol. 2006;194(3):718-21.
14. American Association of Gynecologic Laparoscopists. AAGL practice report: practice guidelines for the diagnosis and management of endometrial polyps. J Minim Invasive Gynecol. 2012;19(1):3-10.
15. Hedrick Ellenson L, Ronnett BM, Kurman RJ. Precursor Lesions of Endometrial Carcinoma. In: Kurman RJ, Hedrick Ellenson L, Ronnett BM (Eds). Blaustein's Pathology of the Female Genital Tract, 6th edition. New York: Springer; 2010.
16. Paramsothy P, Harlow SD, Greendale GA, Gold EB, Crawford SL, Elliott MR, et al. Bleeding patterns during the menopausal transition in the multi-ethnic Study of Women's Health Across the Nation (SWAN): a prospective cohort study. BJOG. 2014;121:1564.
17. Shoff SM, Newcomb PA. Diabetes, body size, and risk of endometrial cancer. Am J Epidemiol. 1998;148:234.
18. Van Hunsel FP, Kampschöer P. Postmenopausal bleeding and dietary supplements: a possible causal relationship with hop- and soy-containing preparations. Ned Tijdschr Geneeskd. 2012;156:A5095.

19. Sabadell J, Castellví J, Baró F. Tuberculous endometritis presenting as postmenopausal bleeding. Int J Gynaecol Obstet. 2007;96:203.
20. Mengistu Z, Engh V, Melby KK, Lippe E, Qvigstad E. Postmenopausal vaginal bleeding caused by endometrial tuberculosis. Acta Obstet Gynecol Scand. 2007;86:631.
21. Güngördük K, Ulker V, Sahbaz A, Ark C, Tekirdag AI. Postmenopausal tuberculosis endometritis. Infect Dis Obstet Gynecol. 2007;2007:27028.
22. American College of Obstetricians and Gynecologists. ACOG Committee Opinion No. 440: the Role of Transvaginal Ultrasonography in the Evaluation of Postmenopausal Bleeding. Obstet Gynecol. 2009;114:4.
23. Goldstein SR, Nachtigall M, Snyder JR, Nachtigall L. Endometrial assessment by vaginal ultrasonography before endometrial sampling in patients with postmenopausal bleeding. Am J Obstet Gynecol. 1990;163:119-23.
24. Varner RE, Sparks JM, Cameron CD, Roberts LL, Soong SJ. Transvaginal sonography of the endometrium in postmenopausal women. Obstet Gynecol. 1991;78:195-9.
25. Granberg S, Wikland M, Karlsson B, Norström A, Friberg LG. Endometrial thickness as measured by endovaginal ultrasonography for identifying endometrial abnormality. Am J Obstet Gynecol. 1991;164:47-52.
26. Gull B, Karlsson B, Milsom I, Granberg S. Can ultrasound replace diltation and curettage? A longitudinal evaluation of postmenopausal bleeding and transvaginal sonographic measurement of the endometrium as predictors of endometrial cancer. Am J Obstet Gynecol. 2003;188:401-8.
27. Epstein E, Ramirez A, Skoog L, Valentin L. Dilatation and curettage fails to detect most focal lesions in the uterine cavity in women with postmenopausal bleeding. Acta Obstet Gynecol Scand. 2001;80:1131.
28. Wang J, Wieslander C, Hansen G, Cass I, Vasilev S, Holschneider CH. Thin endometrial echo complex on ultrasound does not reliably exclude type 2 endometrial cancers. Gynecol Oncol. 2006;101:120.
29. Chandavarkar U, Kuperman J, Muderspach L, Yessaian A, Pham HQ, Lin Y, et al. Postmenopausal endometrial cancer: Reevaluating the role of endometrial echo complex. Gynecol Oncol. 2011;120:S11.
30. SEER. (2011). Cander: CSR 1975-2007. [online] Available from: http://seer.cancer.gov/csr/1975_2007/browse_csr.php?section=5&page=sect_05_table.07.html [Last accessed March, 2021].
31. Partridge EE, Abu-Rustum NR, Campos SM, Fahey PJ, Farmer M, Garcia RL, et al. Cervical cancer screening. J Natl Compr Canc Netw. 2010;8:1358.
32. Rosen MW, Tasset J, Kobernik EK, Smith YR, Johnston C, Quint EH. Risk Factors for Endometrial Cancer or Hyperplasia in Adolescents and Women 25 Years Old or Younger. J Pediatr Adolesc Gynecol. 2019;32:546.
33. Vetter MH, Smith B, Benedict J, Hade EM, Bixel K, Copeland LJ, et al. Preoperative predictors of endometrial cancer at time of hysterectomy for endometrial intraepithelial neoplasia or complex atypical hyperplasia. Am J Obstet Gynecol. 2020;222:60.e1.
34. Karlsson B, Granberg S, Wikland M, Ylöstalo P, Torvid K, Marsal K, et al. Transvaginal ultrasonography of the endometrium in women with postmenopausal bleeding—a Nordic multicenter study. Am J Obstet Gynecol. 1995;172:1488.
35. Emons G, Beckmann MW, Schmidt D, Mallmann P; Uterus commission of the Gynecological Oncology Working Group (AGO). New WHO Classification of Endometrial Hyperplasias. Geburtshilfe Frauenheilkd. 2015;75:135-6.
36. Gallos ID, Shehmar M, Thangaratinam S, Papapostolou TK, Coomarasamy A, Gupta JK. Oral progestogens vs levonorgestrel-releasing intrauterine system for endometrial hyperplasia: a systematic review and meta-analysis. Am J Obstet Gynecol. 2010;203:547.e1.

37. Abu Hashim H, Ghayaty E, El Rakhawy M. Levonorgestrel-releasing intrauterine system vs oral progestins for non-atypical endometrial hyperplasia: a systematic review and metaanalysis of randomized trials. Am J Obstet Gynecol. 2015;213:469.
38. Rakha E, Wong SC, Soomro I, Chaudry Z, Sharma A, Deen S, et al. Clinical outcome of atypical endometrial hyperplasia diagnosed on an endometrial biopsy: institutional experience and review of literature. Am J Surg Pathol. 2012;36:1683.
39. Reed SD, Newton KM, Garcia RL, Allison KH, Voigt LF, Jordan CD, et al. Complex hyperplasia with and without atypia: clinical outcomes and implications of progestin therapy. Obstet Gynecol. 2010;116:365.
40. Gunderson CC, Fader AN, Carson KA, Bristow RE. Oncologic and reproductive outcomes with progestin therapy in women with endometrial hyperplasia and grade 1 adenocarcinoma: a systematic review. Gynecol Oncol. 2012;125:477.
41. Gallos ID, Krishan P, Shehmar M, Ganesan R, Gupta JK. Relapse of endometrial hyperplasia after conservative treatment: a cohort study with long-term follow-up. Hum Reprod. 2013;28:1231.
42. Suckling JA, Kennedy R, Lethaby A. Local oestrogen for vaginal atrophy in postmenopausal women. Cochrane Database of Syst Rev. 2006;(4):CD001500.

Risk and Benefits of Menopausal Hormone Therapy

CHAPTER 16

■ INTRODUCTION

Menopausal hormone therapy (MHT) use in women is constantly evolving. In the last decade, after the women's health initiative (WHI) results, prescription of MHT has been challenging for providers caring for menopausal women. Today fear, uncertainty and anxiety regarding MHT, has been replaced by some clarity about the risks and benefits of MHT. Most of the guidelines and the Endocrine/Menopause Societies agree that MHT is indicated for the management of menopausal symptoms but not for the primary prevention of chronic diseases such as cardiovascular disease (CVD), osteoporosis, or dementia.[1-4] The benefits of MHT appear to outweigh its risks for most symptomatic women who are either under 60 years or less than 10 years from menopause.[5] This timing is referred as timing hypothesis or window opportunity. In older women and women more than 60 years or 10 years after the final menstrual period, the risks benefits balance of MHT is less favorable particularly with regard to cardiovascular risk and cognitive impairment.

While the WHI study clearly demonstrated the adverse effects of MHT in older postmenopausal women (over age 60 years), this is not the age group that presents with new onset of menopausal symptoms. Almost all women who seek medical therapy for menopausal symptoms do so in their late 40s or 50s.

Many expert groups do suggest MHT for younger postmenopausal women with moderate-to-severe symptoms and having no contraindications to estrogen use.[1,3,4] In the past, some experts advised that MHT be limited to 5 years of use. However, hot flushes can last for a decade or more in many women. Therefore, International Menopause Society (IMS) suggested that longer therapy is reasonable in selected women with persistent symptoms. In that case, reassessment, evaluation and further counseling are necessary. Benefits of MHT was assessed by the study in USA which showed:

- "A USD 4.1 billion increase in expenditure for excess chronic diseases {37,549 excess events [breast cancer, coronary heart disease (CHD), colon cancer, fractures]} among women in their 50s and more after stopping the menopause hormone therapy since result of WHI published in 2002.
- In a second analysis of the impact of avoiding unopposed estrogen therapy post-WHI (women post-hysterectomy), an important increase in mortality rates in women ages 50–59 years was calculated (a minimum of 18,601 and as many as 91,601 additional deaths)."[6,14]

■ RESULT OF USE OF MHT FROM WOMEN'S HEALTH INITIATIVE

As noted earlier, the WHI demonstrated adverse effects of MHT in older postmenopausal women (over age 60 years or more than 10 years since menopause); this is not the age group that presents with new onset of menopausal symptoms. Almost all women who seek medical therapy for menopausal symptoms do so in their late 40s or 50s. When counseling symptomatic women considering hormone therapy (HT), the clinician should provide the best estimate of potential risks and benefits for 5 years of use based upon data from women in their 50s.[1] But it is important to mention that duration of MHT could be longer if really necessary.

Although most available HT clinical trial data are from women over age 60 years, estimates of the absolute risks and benefits for women starting MHT in their 50s have been published.[7,8] The intervention phase of the WHI was the source of data for the analysis. Data were expressed as the attributable excess risk or benefit for 5 years of combined estrogen-progestin or unopposed estrogen use in women starting treatment in later age from menopause. Overall, the risk-benefit profile was more favorable for women ages 50–59 compared with older women.[8] We may see the effects from following discussion.

Combined estrogen-progestin therapy: Number of cases (additional or fewer) per 1,000 women per 5 years of hormone use when compared with placebo:
- *CHD*: 2.5 additional cases
- *Invasive breast cancer*: 3 additional cases
- *Stroke*: 2.5 additional cases
- *Pulmonary embolism*: 3 additional cases
- *Colorectal cancer*: 0.5 fewer cases
- *Endometrial cancer*: No difference
- *Hip fracture*: 1.5 fewer cases
- *All-cause mortality*: 5 fewer events.

Estrogen-alone therapy: Number of cases (additional or fewer) per 1,000 women per 5 years of hormone use when compared with placebo:
- *CHD*: 5.5 fewer cases
- *Invasive breast cancer*: 2.5 fewer cases
- *Stroke*: 0.5 fewer cases
- *Pulmonary embolism*: 1.5 additional cases
- *Colorectal cancer*: 0.5 fewer cases
- *Hip fracture*: 1.5 additional cases (of note, there was an overall decrease in all osteoporotic fractures in both the estrogen and combined estrogen-progestin groups)
- *All-cause mortality*: 5.5 fewer events.

This analysis highlights that the overall risks of MHT in younger postmenopausal women are considerably lower than those for older women (e.g., women in the WHI). The major explanation for the difference in absolute excess risk between older and younger postmenopausal women is the lower baseline risk of CHD, stroke, venous thromboembolism (VTE), and breast cancer in younger postmenopausal women.[7,8]

A subgroup analysis of a 10-year MHT trial for osteoporosis [Danish Osteoporosis Prevention Study (DOPS)] reported that women taking MHT had a reduced risk of the composite outcome of mortality, heart failure, or myocardial infarction, without an increased risk of stroke, VTE, or cancer.[9]

■ RESULT OF RECENT STUDIES

Withholding MHT from symptomatic women might pose a risk, particularly with regard to CVD and osteoporosis. Estrogen use after oophorectomy does not increase the risk of breast cancer among women with BRCA1 mutation carriers. The Kronos Early Estrogen Prevention Study (KEEPS), a 4-year, randomized, double-blind, placebo-controlled trial (in women ages 45-54 years), reported that, when combined with cyclical monthly oral progesterone, oral conjugated estrogen (0.45 mg daily) or transdermal estrogen (50 µg daily) reduced menopausal symptoms. Surrogate markers of atherosclerosis [coronary artery calcium and carotid intima-media thickness (CIMT)] were not significantly different in the HT and placebo groups.[10]

In the Early versus Late Intervention Trial with Estradiol (ELITE) study showed, progression of subclinical atherosclerosis (measured as CIMT) was slower than placebo in the early intervention group, while rates of progression were similar to placebo in the late intervention group.[11]

A lower risk of CHD (composite of death from cardiovascular causes and nonfatal myocardial infarction) compared with placebo [relative risk (RR) 0.52, 95% CI 0.29-0.96; eight fewer cases of heart disease per 1,000 women treated per year].

A lower mortality rate [RR 0.70, 95% CI 0.52-0.95; six fewer deaths per 1,000 women treated per year] was most promising findings.

The quality of the evidence from DOPS study for the mortality and CHD meta-analyses was rated as moderate.[9]

Therefore, MHT needs to be individualized for women with CVD if there is indication for MHT, risk assessment of CVD need to be done for the prescription of MH. Risk assessment can be done by taking history, clinical examination and some investigation. American Heart Association prescribes MHT, which is described in **Table 1**.

Stroke: In the WHI, a 31% increase in stroke risk was seen with combined conjugated equine estrogens-medroxyprogesterone acetate use compared with placebo (intention-to-treat HR 1.31, 95% CI 1.02-1.68).[12]

Excess risk was seen in all age groups[13] and was independent of other known risk factors for stroke. In the unopposed estrogen trial, stroke risk was significantly increased with conjugated equine estrogen versus placebo (HR 1.39, 95% CI 1.1-1.77).[14]

TABLE 1: Evaluating CVD risk in women contemplating MHT.

10-year CVD risk	Years since menopause onset <10 years
Low (<5%)	MHT ok
Moderate (5–10%)	MHT ok (choose transdermal)
High (>10)*	Avoid MHT

CVD risk calculated by ACC/AHA cardiovascular risk calculator, methods to calculate risk and risk stratification vary among countries.

Stroke risk appears to be lower with transdermal compared with oral estrogen preparations.

For women ages 50–59 years, the estimates of excess VTE risk was seen, 1.3 additional cases per 1,000 women per 5 years of combined estrogen-progestin or unopposed estrogen use.[8]

The risk of VTE appears to be lower with transdermal compared with oral estrogen preparations. In addition, risk may vary by type of progestin.

■ MORTALITY

Younger menopausal women (ages 50–59) may actually have a reduction in all-cause mortality with MHT.[15]

In an earlier analysis, women ages 50–59 years, the group most likely to be taking HT, the estimate of mortality benefit in one analysis was 5.3 and 5 fewer deaths per 1,000 per 5 years of combined estrogen-progestin or unopposed estrogen use, respectively.[8]

Breast cancer: In the WHI, the risk of invasive breast cancer was significantly increased with combined HT at an average follow-up of 5.6 years [hazard ratio (HR) 1.24, unadjusted 95% CI 1.01–1.54].[16]

In contrast to the results of the combined HT trial, a trend toward a lower rate of breast cancer risk was seen in the unopposed estrogen trial (HR 0.77 for unopposed estrogen vs. placebo, 95% CI 0.59–1.01).[7]

Current MHT regimens typically include lower doses of estrogen as well as a different type and route [e.g., transdermal 17-beta estradiol (17-beta-E2)], with micronized progesterone, which is now considered the progestin of choice by most experts.[1,3,4] It is thought that transdermal 17-beta-E2 and micronized progesterone is associated with lower breast cancer risk than conjugated estrogens and medroxyprogesterone acetate combination. Progesterone choice is critical regarding breast cancer. Natural progesterone and dihydrogesterne have much safety profile than medroxyprogesterone.

Ovarian cancer: A meta-analysis of 52 epidemiologic studies including 21,488 postmenopausal women with ovarian cancer suggests that there is a small excess risk of ovarian cancer with MHT use.[17] Ovarian cancer risk was greater in ever-users versus never-users of MHT (RR 1.14, 95% CI 1.10–1.19). Risks were similar for estrogen-only and estrogen-progestin users. The calculated absolute excess risk associated with MHT was very low; 5 years of MHT use in women ages 50–54 years would result in approximately one additional ovarian cancer case per 1,000 users.

Endometrial hyperplasia and carcinoma: Treatment of postmenopausal women with estrogen alone increases the risk of endometrial hyperplasia and carcinoma.[18] Within 1 year, endometrial hyperplasia can be demonstrated in 20–50% of women receiving unopposed estrogen.[19,20] Furthermore, studies have shown an increased incidence of endometrial carcinoma with long-term unopposed estrogen, with the RR ranging from 3.1 to 15. The risk of endometrial hyperplasia and cancer with unopposed estrogen therapy is both duration and dose dependent.

Protective effect of progestins: As noted in the WHI, among women treated with estrogen, the excess risk of endometrial hyperplasia and carcinoma can be largely abolished by concurrent therapy with a progestin given in either a cyclic or continuous regimen.[21-23]

In the PEPI trial and in a review from the Cochrane Database, cyclic progestin (when given at least 12 days per month) was as effective as continuous low-dose progestin.[24] Shorter-duration progestin therapy (<10 days) may be less protective.[25-28] Cyclic monthly users of estrogen-progestin had a higher risk of endometrial cancer than continuous estrogen-progestin users.[29]

A commonly used combined continuous estrogen-progestin regimen has low-dose medroxyprogesterone (2.5 or 5 mg daily) given each day with estrogen (conjugated estrogens 0.625 mg or its equivalent). This regimen is associated with a low risk of endometrial hyperplasia[30] and has the added advantage of inducing amenorrhea in 60–75% of women after more than 6 months of treatment.[31,32]

Other estrogen-progestin regimens that have been investigated include the following and very promising:
- Oral micronized progesterone (200 mg/day for 12 days) reduces the risk of hyperplasia to the same degree as medroxyprogesterone acetate (2.5 mg/day continuously or 10 mg/day for 12 days).[33]
- Medroxyprogesterone (10 mg/day) for 14 days every 3 months may be associated with higher than normal rates of endometrial hyperplasia and cannot be recommended.[34,35]
- Lower doses of combined estrogen-progestin therapy [conjugated estrogen (0.3 or 0.45 mg/day) with medroxyprogesterone acetate (1.5 or 2.5 mg/day)] also appear to be endometrial protective.[36]
- Levonorgestrel-releasing intrauterine systems (LNG-IUS) are contraceptive agents that have been used for endometrial protection by some peri- and postmenopausal women taking estrogen. The strategy is to avoid the potential excess risk of CVD and breast cancer associated with systemic therapy.

Colorectal cancer: In the WHI, the risk of colorectal cancer was reduced with combined conjugated equine estrogens-medroxyprogesterone acetate use (43 vs. 72 cases in the hormone and placebo groups, respectively; HR 0.56, 95% CI 0.38-0.81).[37]

Both unopposed estrogen and combined estrogen-progestin therapy had no global cognitive benefits. Neither type of MHT prevented dementia in older, nondemented postmenopausal women; on the contrary, it increased risk.

The risk of osteoporotic fracture with combined HT vs. placebo was reduced at the hip (HR 0.67, unadjusted 95% CI 0.47-0.96) and at the vertebrae and wrist (HR 0.65, unadjusted 95% CI 0.46-0.92 and HR 0.71, 95% CI 0.59-0.85, respectively).[38]

Combined MHT appears to reduce the risk of type 2 diabetes mellitus, possibly mediated by a decrease in insulin resistance unrelated to body size. However, this effect is insufficient to recommend MHT as a diabetes prevention strategy in women with CHD.

Estrogen therapy, in particular, vaginal estrogen, is effective for the symptoms of genitourinary syndrome of menopause. Estrogen may also be beneficial for reducing the frequency of recurrent urinary tract infections in postmenopausal women, but the effect appears to be specific to vaginal estrogen, as illustrated by the following studies: A randomized controlled trial found that vaginal estrogen decreased the risk of recurrence in patients with frequent urinary tract infections (0.5 vs. 5.9 episodes per patient-year).[39]

Health-related quality-of-life: Estrogen has a variable effect on quality-of-life in postmenopausal women, depending on the women's age and the presence of symptoms and/or comorbid conditions. In postmenopausal women with vasomotor flushes, estrogen appears to improve quality-of-life.[40,41]

Osteoporosis and falls: Problems with balance may play a major role in the incidence of forearm fractures in postmenopausal women.[42] Estrogen therapy may improve balance and reduce the tendency to fall, a change that could contribute to the associated decrease in fracture risk. Some studies have noted an improvement in balance with estrogen therapy.[43] MHT prevents early bone loss and reduces fractures in postmenopausal women. Long-term MHT use in the indication of bone preservation is considered an option for women having high risks of osteoporotic fracture, particularly when other products have been poorly tolerated, are contraindicated, or have unfavorable risk benefit balance.

Eyes: Dry eye disease (DED) is thought to be related in part to estrogen deficiency; its rates in women increase after menopause.[44]

However, in a meta-analysis of nine clinical trials in women with DED, improvements were seen in the symptoms of dryness, foreign body sensation, and burning compared with controls MHT may also reduce intraocular pressure and lower the risk of primary open-angle glaucoma[45] but the absolute reduction in risk is small.

Weight: Although women are often concerned that taking MHT will exacerbate the weight gain that occurs in midlife, a meta-analysis of 28 trials in 28,559 women found no evidence of an effect of unopposed estrogen or combined estrogen-progestin on body weight or body mass index.[46]

WOMEN WITH PRIMARY OVARIAN INSUFFICIENCY (PREMATURE OVARIAN FAILURE)

Menopausal hormone therapy is generally initiated at a younger age. In otherwise healthy women with primary ovarian insufficiency, they should continue their MHT until the average age of menopause, approximately age 50–51 years. After that continuation of MHT is possible if indicated and with optimum counseling.

KEY MESSAGES

- Menopausal hormone therapy if administered for clear indication with in the 10 years of menopause or in women aged below 60 years, its benefits outweigh the risks.
- MHT improves vasomotor symptoms, vulvovaginal atrophy/GSM, the quality life of menopause women. It decreases new onset of type 2 diabetes, metabolic syndrome, cardiovascular mortality, enhances sexual function and prevents osteoporotic bone loss.
- To get maximum benefits and minimum side effects, MHT needs to start with lowest dose.
- It can be used for 5 years without any adverse effects. But it can be used longer if indicated with reassessment and proper counseling. So duration of MHT depends on patient's profile or individualization.
- MHT reduces all causes of mortality, relieves menopausal symptoms effectively, and reduces colorectal cancer.
- MHT is the choice of drug for relief of vasomotor symptoms, genitourinary symptoms of menopause and it prevents bone loss.
- Absolute risk of breast cancer is low, but still better to avoid in women having strong breast cancer risk. Right choice of the type of MHT is critical. Choice of progestin is important, safety profile of micronized progesterone and that of dihydrogesterone are better.
- Endometrial cancer by unopposed estrogen can be prevented by addition of optimum dose of progesterone.
- Risk of thromboembolism of oral estrogen can be minimized by transdermal estrogen, which bypasses the hepatic metabolism.
- Proper counseling is cornerstone to achieve benefits from MHT, right selection of MHT and mode of delivery after individualization avoids the risks of MHT.

- It is advocated that these subsets of women with premature menopause need to be counseled for shared decision-making on the ideal dose and duration of MHT, using the best available information on safety and efficacy.

REFERENCES

1. Mosca L, Benjamin EJ, Berra K, Bezanson JL, Dolor RJ, Lloyd-Jones DM, et al. Effectiveness-based guidelines for the prevention of cardiovascular disease in women—2011 update: a guideline from the American Heart Association. Circulation. 2011;123:1243-6.
2. ACOG Practice Bulletin No. 141: management of menopausal symptoms. Obstet Gynecol. 2014;123:202. Reaffirmed 2018.
3. The NAMS 2017 Hormone Therapy Position Statement Advisory Panel. The 2017 hormone therapy position statement of The North American Menopause Society. Menopause. 2017;24:728.
4. US Preventive Services Task Force, Grossman DC, Curry SJ, Owens DK, Barry MJ, Davidson KW, et al. Hormone Therapy for the Primary Prevention of Chronic Conditions in Postmenopausal Women: US Preventive Services Task Force Recommendation Statement. JAMA. 2017;318:2224-33.
5. Stuenkel CA, Davis SR, Gompel A, Lumsden MA, Murad MH, Pinkerton JV, et al. Treatment of Symptoms of the Menopause: An Endocrine Society Clinical Practice Guideline. J Clin Endocrinol Metab. 2015;100:3975.
6. Sarrel PM, Njike VY, Vinante V, Katz DL. The mortality toll of estrogen avoidance: an analysis of excess deaths among hysterectomized women aged 50 to 59 years. Am J Public Health. 2013;103:1583.
7. Manson JE, Chlebowski RT, Stefanick ML, Aragaki AK, Rossouw JE, Prentice RL, et al. Menopausal hormone therapy and health outcomes during the intervention and extended poststopping phases of the Women's Health Initiative randomized trials. JAMA. 2013;310:1353.
8. Santen RJ, Allred DC, Ardoin SP, Archer DF, Boyd N, Braunstein GD, et al. Postmenopausal hormone therapy: an Endocrine Society scientific statement. J Clin Endocrinol Metab. 2010;95:s1.
9. Schierbeck LL, Rejnmark L, Tofteng CL, Stilgren L, Eiken P, Mosekilde L, et al. Effect of hormone replacement therapy on cardiovascular events in recently postmenopausal women: randomised trial. BMJ. 2012;345:e6409.
10. Harman SM, Black DM, Naftolin F, Brinton EA, Budoff MJ, Cedars MI, et al. Arterial imaging outcomes and cardiovascular risk factors in recently menopausal women: a randomized trial. Ann Intern Med. 2014;161:249.
11. Hodis HN, Mack WJ, Henderson VW, Shoupe D, Budoff MJ, Hwang-Levine J, et al. Vascular Effects of Early versus Late Postmenopausal Treatment with Estradiol. N Engl J Med. 2016;374:1221.
12. Wassertheil-Smoller S, Hendrix SL, Limacher M, Heiss G, Kooperberg C, Baird A, et al. Effect of estrogen plus progestin on stroke in postmenopausal women: the Women's Health Initiative: a randomized trial. JAMA. 2003;289:2673.
13. Rossouw JE, Prentice RL, Manson JE, Wu L, Barad D, Barnabei VM, et al. Postmenopausal hormone therapy and risk of cardiovascular disease by age and years since menopause. JAMA. 2007;297:1465-77.
14. Anderson GL, Limacher M, Assaf AR, Bassford T, Beresford SA, Black H, et al. Effects of conjugated equine estrogen in postmenopausal women with hysterectomy: the Women's Health Initiative randomized controlled trial. JAMA. 2004;291:1701-12.
15. Manson JE, Aragaki AK, Rossouw JE, Anderson GL, Prentice RL, LaCroix AZ, et al. Menopausal Hormone Therapy and Long-term All-Cause and Cause-Specific Mortality: the Women's Health Initiative Randomized Trials. JAMA. 2017;318:927-38.

16. Chlebowski RT, Hendrix SL, Langer RD, Stefanick ML, Gass M, Lane D, et al. Influence of estrogen plus progestin on breast cancer and mammography in healthy postmenopausal women: the Women's Health Initiative Randomized Trial. JAMA. 2003;289:3243-53.
17. Collaborative Group On Epidemiological Studies Of Ovarian Cancer, Beral V, Gaitskell K, Hermon C, Moser K, Reeves G, et al. Menopausal hormone use and ovarian cancer risk: individual participant meta-analysis of 52 epidemiological studies. Lancet. 2015;385:1835.
18. Beral V, Bull D, Reeves G, Million Women Study Collaborators. Endometrial cancer and hormone-replacement therapy in the Million Women Study. Lancet. 2005;365:1543.
19. Woodruff JD, Pickar JH. Incidence of endometrial hyperplasia in postmenopausal women taking conjugated estrogens (Premarin) with medroxyprogesterone acetate or conjugated estrogens alone. The Menopause Study Group. Am J Obstet Gynecol. 1994;170:1213.
20. Schiff I, Sela HK, Cramer D, Tulchinsky D, Ryan KJ. Endometrial hyperplasia in women on cyclic or continuous estrogen regimens. Fertil Steril. 1982;37:79-82.
21. Beresford SA, Weiss NS, Voigt LF, McKnight B. Risk of endometrial cancer in relation to use of oestrogen combined with cyclic progestagen therapy in postmenopausal women. Lancet. 1997;349:458-61.
22. Effects of hormone replacement therapy on endometrial histology in postmenopausal women. The Postmenopausal Estrogen/Progestin Interventions (PEPI) Trial. The Writing Group for the PEPI Trial. JAMA. 1996;275:370.
23. Lacey JV Jr, Leitzmann MF, Chang SC, Mouw T, Hollenbeck AR, Schatzkin A, et al. Endometrial cancer and menopausal hormone therapy in the National Institutes of Health-AARP Diet and Health Study cohort. Cancer. 2007;109:1303.
24. Furness S, Roberts H, Marjoribanks J, Lethaby A. Hormone therapy in postmenopausal women and risk of endometrial hyperplasia. Cochrane Database Syst Rev. 2012:CD000402.
25. Pike MC, Peters RK, Cozen W, Probst-Hensch NM, Felix JC, Wan PC, et al. Estrogen-progestin replacement therapy and endometrial cancer. J Natl Cancer Inst. 1997;89:1110-6.
26. Cerin A, Heldaas K, Moeller B. Adverse endometrial effects of long-cycle estrogen and progestogen replacement therapy. The Scandinavian LongCycle Study Group. N Engl J Med. 1996;334:668.
27. Whitehead MI, Fraser D. The effects of estrogens and progestogens on the endometrium. Modern approach to treatment. Obstet Gynecol Clin North Am. 1987;14:299.
28. Whitehead MI, Hillard TC, Crook D. The role and use of progestogens. Obstet Gynecol. 1990;75:59S.
29. Jaakkola S, Lyytinen H, Pukkala E, Ylikorkala O. Endometrial cancer in postmenopausal women using estradiol-progestin therapy. Obstet Gynecol. 2009;114:1197.
30. Weinstein L, Bewtra C, Gallagher JC. Evaluation of a continuous combined low-dose regimen of estrogen-progestin for treatment of the menopausal patient. Am J Obstet Gynecol. 1990;162:1534.
31. Archer DF, Pickar JH, Bottiglioni F. Bleeding patterns in postmenopausal women taking continuous combined or sequential regimens of conjugated estrogens with medroxyprogesterone acetate. Menopause Study Group. Obstet Gynecol. 1994;83:686.
32. Creasman WT, Henderson D, Hinshaw W, Clarke-Pearson DL. Estrogen replacement therapy in the patient treated for endometrial cancer. Obstet Gynecol. 1986;67:326.
33. Effects of estrogen or estrogen/progestin regimens on heart disease risk factors in postmenopausal women. The Postmenopausal Estrogen/Progestin Interventions (PEPI) Trial. The Writing Group for the PEPI Trial. JAMA. 1995;273:199.

34. Ettinger B, Selby J, Citron JT, Vangessel A, Ettinger VM, Hendrickson MR. Cyclic hormone replacement therapy using quarterly progestin. Obstet Gynecol. 1994; 83:693-700.
35. Hirvonen E, Salmi T, Puolakka J, Heikkinen J, Granfors E, Hulkko S, et al. Can progestin be limited to every third month only in postmenopausal women taking estrogen? Maturitas. 1995;21:39.
36. Pickar JH, Yeh IT, Wheeler JE, Cunnane MF, Speroff L. Endometrial effects of lower doses of conjugated equine estrogens and medroxyprogesterone acetate: two-year substudy results. Fertil Steril. 2003;80:1234-40.
37. Chlebowski RT, Wactawski-Wende J, Ritenbaugh C, Hubbell FA, Ascensao J, Rodabough RJ, et al. Estrogen plus progestin and colorectal cancer in postmenopausal women. N Engl J Med. 2004;350:991-1004.
38. Cauley JA, Robbins J, Chen Z, Cummings SR, Jackson RD, LaCroix AZ, et al. Effects of estrogen plus progestin on risk of fracture and bone mineral density: the Women's Health Initiative randomized trial. JAMA. 2003;290:1729-38.
39. Raz R, Stamm WE. A controlled trial of intravaginal estriol in postmenopausal women with recurrent urinary tract infections. N Engl J Med. 1993;329:753.
40. MacLennan A, Lester S, Moore V. Oral estrogen replacement therapy versus placebo for hot flushes: a systematic review. Climacteric. 2001;4:58.
41. Col NF, Weber G, Stiggelbout A, Chuo J, D'Agostino R, Corso P. Short-term menopausal hormone therapy for symptom relief: an updated decision model. Arch Intern Med. 2004;164:1634-40.
42. Ekblad S, Bergendahl A, Enler P, Ledin T, Möllen C, Hammar M. Disturbances in postural balance are common in postmenopausal women with vasomotor symptoms. Climacteric. 2000;3:192-8.
43. Hammar ML, Lindgren R, Berg GE, Möller CG, Niklasson MK. Effects of hormonal replacement therapy on the postural balance among postmenopausal women. Obstet Gynecol. 1996; 88:955-60.
44. Sullivan DA, Rocha EM, Aragona P, Clayton JA, Ding J, Golebiowski B, et al. TFOS DEWS II Sex, Gender, and Hormones Report. Ocul Surf. 2017;15:284.
45. Norman RJ, Flight IH, Rees MC. Oestrogen and progestogen hormone replacement therapy for peri-menopausal and post-menopausal women: weight and body fat distribution. Cochrane Database Syst Rev. 2000:CD001018.
46. Newman-Casey PA, Talwar N, Nan B, Musch DC, Pasquale LR, Stein JD. The potential association between postmenopausal hormone use and primary open-angle glaucoma. JAMA Ophthalmol. 2014;132:298-303.

CHAPTER 17
Prescribing Hormone Replacement Therapy

■ INTRODUCTION

The constantly changing landscape regarding menopausal hormone therapy (MHT) has been challenging for providers caring for menopausal women. Age and time since menopause affect the balance of benefits and risks for hormone therapy used in postmenopausal women. Since the Women's Health Initiative (WHI) 2002, women and the healthcare providers are scared to prescribe MHT in era of breast cancer and cardiovascular diseases (CVD). But those findings were reanalyzed and revisited and found that the study was biased where most women were included who were aged more than 60 years who had already some diseases. The study included only one dose of estrogen and only one kind of progesterone medroxyprogesterone acetate (MPA) that did not reflect the whole truth of MHT.

Most recent studies showed that for healthy women experiencing menopausal symptoms around the average age of natural menopause, MHT provides excellent symptom relief and poses low risk. Withholding MHT from symptomatic women might pose a risk, particularly with regard to cardiovascular disease and osteoporosis.

Since a large proportion of menopausal women will suffer the consequences of cardiovascular disease and osteoporosis, the role of MHT in ameliorating these debilitating conditions need to be considered.

MHT may be associated with increased risk when initiated in older women and is generally avoided. But the global consensus is that women suffering from primary ovarian insufficiency (POI) should use MHT continuously up to the age of menopause to improve the quality-of-life and/or prevention of adverse consequences of deficiency of estrogen. For symptomatic menopausal women who are under 60 years of age or within 10 years of menopause, the benefits of MHT generally outweigh the risks. The "timing hypothesis" suggests that starting hormone therapy early in menopause (compared with starting it 10 years or more after the onset of menopause) may be cardioprotective because of estrogen's apparent ability to slow the progression of atherosclerosis in younger women.[1,2] Although the evidence suggests that beginning hormone therapy near the start of menopause decreases the risk of cardiac disease, further study is needed.

Current guidelines recommend against using hormone therapy to prevent or treat cardiac disease.[3] Further, the American Academy of Family Physicians recommends against using hormone therapy for the prevention of chronic conditions.[4]

Systemic MHT initiated early in menopause appears to slow the progression of atherosclerotic disease, thereby reducing the risk of cardiovascular disease and mortality.

Updated guidelines for MHT use have been provided by the North American Menopause Society, European Menopause Society, British Menopause Society, and multiple others, with consensus statements incorporating this concept issued in 2012 and 2013, will be discussed below that will guide to prescribe right MHT for right women.

The science of MHT is evolving, and it is important to stay informed and keep an open perspective as our understanding about these agents improves.

■ EVALUATION FOR THE PRESCRIPTION

Thorough assessment with detail medical history and clinical examination should be done. Aim to assess the need or clear indication of hormone therapy ant to assess any risk factors that do not favor MHT. History taking involves finding out issues in symptomatic women and to find out any risk factors for MHT.

Gynecological history: Current menstrual status, age at menopause, last menstrual period, flow pattern before menopause, and contraception.

Obstetric history: Numbers of pregnancies, miscarriages, living issues, lactation, postpartum depression, history of gestational diabetes, hypertension.

Medical diseases: Any medical diseases.

Surgical history: Any surgery, thyroid, breast uterus, ovaries.

Family history of chronic illness such as DM, hypertension, heart diseases, migraine, cancer, stroke, early menopause, osteoporosis, Alzheimer's disease, rheumatoid, and thyroid disease.

Personal history: About diet, level of physical activity, mental attitude, social relationship, habits, mood changes, memory and concentration, and use of caffeine, tobacco, alcohol, details about bowel, bladder habit, and sexual history.

Clinical examination includes:
- Height, weight, body mass index, waist circumference
- Pulse, blood pressure, edema
- Auscultation of heart and lung
- Breast examination
- Per-abdominal examination
- Pelvic examination
- Eye checkup, dental checkup
- Spine, muscle mass and strength, and varicose vein.

Menopause hormone therapy involves the administration of synthetic estrogen and progestogen to replace a woman's depleting hormone levels and thus alleviate menopausal symptoms. However, MHT has been linked to various risks; debate regarding its risk-benefit ratio continues. Before prescribing we should follow: First step is to address the reasons why a woman might present, i.e., her symptoms or concerns. Then followed with the menopause staging or the age, and assess them who may have amenorrhea due to hysterectomy, endometrial ablation, or hormonal contraception. MHT can then be recommended to women who are at the right age, have no contraindications, and have low cardiovascular and breast cancer risks. After taking a basic medical history and clinical examination, minimum baseline laboratory and imaging studies should be done before administering HT include the following:

- Hemography, complete blood count
- Urinalysis
- Fasting lipid profile
- Blood sugar profile
- Serum thyroid profile
- Urine and stool routine test
- *Ultrasonography*: To measure endometrial thickness and ovarian volume
- Papanicolaou test
- Mammography/sonogram
- DEXA and electrocardiography, If indicated
- *Mammography*: Performed once every 2–3 years and annually after the age of 50 years.

Checking levels of estradiol, progesterone, and follicle-stimulating hormone is not necessary and generally provides no meaningful information. But risk assessment of CVD, osteoporosis, breast cancer need to be done.

Endometrial sampling is not required in routine practice. However, the presence of abnormal bleeding before or during HT should prompt consideration of ultrasonography to check endometrial thickness (cutoff, <4 mm). If she also complains of spotting then outpatient Pipelle sampling or hysteroscopy can be done. Hysteroscopy is the best investigation but if not feasible, dilation and curettage under general anesthesia is advised.

Reviewing the menopausal symptoms and their possible solutions, including a discussion on lifestyle modifications and MHT, is to be done.

We may go through the following steps before prescribing the MHT.

■ ASSESSMENT OF PATIENT CRITERIA

Is She at the Window of Opportunity?

Age less than 60 years or less than 10 years since her last menstrual period is considered the window of opportunity for initiating MHT. Data from WHI trial showed that if MHT is initiated after 60, it increases the risk of a heart attack and breast cancer.[5] If transdermal hormones containing estradiol and micronized progesterone initiated within the window of opportunity, it is more likely to be protective against cardiovascular disease, bone loss (FDA approved). Therefore, window opportunity is the optimum timing to prescribe MHT.

Rule Out Contraindications for MHT

There are some absolute contraindications for MHT such as unexplained vaginal bleeding, stroke, myocardial infarction (MI), pulmonary embolism (PE), venous thromboembolism (VTE), breast or endometrial cancer, and active liver disease.

Relative contraindications include uncontrolled diabetes, hypertriglyceridemia, active gallbladder disease, CVD, and migraine with aura. If contraindications are present, we need to consider other options. If none, we should go to the next step.

Evaluate Cardiovascular Risk

There are many tools to calculate the CVD risk in a women. History is the most important but also we may follow guideline such as the American College of Cardiology (ACC)/American Heart Association (AHA) 10-year CVD risk (Framingham and Reynolds) or North American Menopause Society NAMS App called MenoPro.[6] It has been validated in women over 45 years with menopausal symptoms. One should follow the local guideline. If national or local guideline is not available, simply we may take detail history focusing any factor pointing the woman for heart disease. To reinforce the findings we may do some investigations for risk assessment of CVD. Total cholesterol value is important. Normal blood pressure measurement goes in favor of good heart health. If the assessment indicates a higher risk of CVD than normal, we need to consider other options to relieve symptoms but not MHT. For medium risk women, we may consider transdermal estrogen instead of oral MHT. If low risk or no risk, we may move to the next step.

Evaluate of Breast Cancer Risk

History of breast cancer in family or personal is most important. Breast cancer risk assessment tool (either national or international) need to followed.[7] Breast examination needs to be done. Mammography need to be done if indicated. If breast cancer risk is apparent we should consider other options. For medium-risk women, caution on MHT is advised. If the risk of breast seems nil or low we may move to the next step.

Uterus Present?

If the answer is yes, estrogen hormone must be added with progesterone while prescribing MHT. If the answer is no, then estrogen alone is sufficient for the majority of women. Women get all the benefits of estrogen therapy.[8]

All the international organizations support the use of MHT for the shortest period, (usually 3–5 years) and the lowest possible dose (of estrogen). After 5 years, the patient should be assessed and if necessary MHT may be continued if indicated after appropriate assessment and counseling. It is not mandatory to stop MHT after 5 years.

The US Task Force for Disease Prevention collected data about the long-term administration of MHT, which seemed MHT ameliorates menopausal symptoms effectively but it is not necessary to use to prevent the incidence of chronic diseases such as osteoporosis, cardiovascular disease and dementia that may be linked to the low estrogenic environment after menopause. At present MHT is indicated only for symptomatic women that is, women are complaining of vasomotor symptoms, low mood, vulvovaginal atrophy, or genitourinary syndrome of menopause. So once decision is taken to prescribe estrogen plus progesterone, next step is following.

Is the Patient on Adequate Doses of Progesterone?

There is chance of endometrial cancer in women who are on estrogen alone or receiving insufficient doses of progesterone.

Regardless of the dose of estrogen, or the route, certain basic conditions need to be applied for the added progesterone:
- The transdermal absorption of progesterone is erratic, and the progesterone cream is not sufficient for endometrial protection. So they are not recommended.
- Cyclic progestin (when given at least 12 days per month) was as effective as continuous low-dose progestin [shorter-duration progestin therapy (<10 days) may be less protective]. Cyclic monthly users of estrogen-progestin had a higher risk of endometrial cancer than continuous estrogen-progestin users.
- A regimen of combined continuous estrogen-progestin regimen has low-dose medroxyprogesterone (2.5 or 5 mg daily) given each day with estrogen (conjugated estrogens 0.625 mg or its equivalent). This regimen is associated with a low risk of endometrial hyperplasia and has the added advantage of inducing amenorrhea in 60–75% of women after more than 6 months of treatment. However though MPA (Provera) and other synthetic progestogens have a good protective effect for endometrium, but they are likely to have a negative impact on breast cancer risk and metabolic parameters (and hence CVD events).[9]
- Other estrogen-progestin regimens that have been include.
- Oral micronized progesterone (200 mg/day for 12 days) reduces the risk of hyperplasia to the same degree as MPA (2.5 mg/day continuously or 10 mg/day for 12 days).
- Lower doses of combined estrogen-progestin therapy [conjugated estrogen (0.3 or 0.45 mg/day) with MPA (1.5 or 2.5 mg/day)] also appear to be endometrial protective so it can be used.

- Levonorgestrel-releasing intrauterine systems (LNG-IUS) are contraceptive agents that have been used for endometrial protection by some peri- and postmenopausal women taking estrogen. The strategy is to avoid the potential excess risk of cardiovascular disease and breast cancer associated with systemic therapy.

Most uniform regimen recommended—oral or transdermal estrogen in combination with micronized progesterone at 100 mg daily.[10] Or sequential use of 200 mg micronized progesterone 14 days in a month can also be employed.

Women who cannot tolerate 100 mg, they may be offered 50 or 75 mg of micronized progesterone should be offered as they do well with this low dose. A yearly transvaginal ultrasound to measure the thickness of the endometrium (please note that a transabdominal ultrasound is not as accurate) is to be done. Progesterone does not eliminate the risk of endometrial cancer completely.[11] If there is any bleeding, a full gynecological assessment is mandatory.

Before considering the prescription we need to keep some points in our mind such as menopause is the permanent cessation of menstruation in a nonhysterectomized woman. Though the average age of natural menopause has been reported as being at 51.5 years but for hysterectomized women menopause appears 2–3 years earlier than natural age of menopause. The climacteric symptoms may appear in perimenopause years.

The perimenopause is the time from the onset of cycle irregularity through until 12 months after the menstrual period. That could be 3–4 years before final cessation of the period.

Surgical menopause is the removal of both ovaries. POI is cessation of ovarian function before the age of 40 years.

Now once we are ready to prescribe MHT, we need to re-evaluate the proper indications of hormone therapy.

Indications for hormone therapy mostly or symptoms relief but MHT prevents bone loss and CVD for them who are using MHT. However, consensus has been reached regarding the use of HT to relieve symptoms:
- To relieve vasomotor symptoms, palpitation
- To improve urogenital symptoms (long-term therapy is required)
- Women suffering from bone loss
- Women with POI.

▪ MENOPAUSAL HORMONE THERAPY

Since publication of the first of the WHI hormone studies, the use of MHT has raised concerns. In 2013, several international medical societies formulated a "Global Consensus Statement on Menopausal Hormone Therapy."[12]

Several core recommendations are listed in this document, with the first being: "MHT is the most effective treatment for vasomotor symptoms associated with menopause at any age, but benefits are more likely to outweigh risks for symptomatic women before the age of 60 years or within 10 years after menopause." There is general consensus that:

- Endometrial protection with a progestogen is essential in nonhysterectomized women, whereas hysterectomized women should be prescribed estrogen alone.
- Women with premature ovarian insufficiency should be treated with MHT at least until the age of natural menopause.
- Oral estrogen is associated with an increased risk of VTE although the absolute risk is small for women <60 years old. The risk appears to be lower/not at all with transdermal estrogen. Therefore, transdermal estrogen is preferred for women at increased risk of VTE, i.e., smokers and in obese women.
- Breast cancer is a contraindication to the use of MHT but can be individualized.
- The prescription of individually formulated and compounded hormone preparations is not recommended.
- MHT prevents bone loss and fractures in women aged up to 60 years, or within 10 years of menopause.
- Testosterone therapy, given in a dose appropriate for a woman, may improve sexual desire and arousal.
- Oral dehydroepiandrosterone (DHEA) is not effective for the treatment of menopausal vasomotor symptoms (VMS), mood changes, or sexual dysfunction.

The primary use of MHT (estrogen ± progestogen therapy) is to alleviate symptoms of the menopause, namely hot flushes, night sweats, sleep disturbance, arthralgia and vaginal dryness and therefore, improve the quality-of-life of women who, without MHT, find these symptoms intolerable.

For women with an intact uterus, progestogen therapy is taken with estrogen to protect the endometrium of the uterus from over-stimulation by unopposed estrogen.

This can be continuous estrogen with cyclic progestogen for 14 days out of a monthly cycle, or as continuous combined MHT where both the estrogen and progestogen are taken every day.

Cyclic MHT results in scheduled menstrual bleeding after the progestogen is ceased.

Continuous combined MHT results no bleeding in 90% of women after 12 months. Breakthrough bleeding is not uncommon in the first few months of this type of regimen. If breakthrough bleeding is persistent for more than 6 months or prolonged, then investigation of the endometrium is required.

For women who have undergone a hysterectomy, the administration of estrogen therapy alone is appropriate.

Menopausal Hormone Therapy Formulations

Menopausal hormone therapy can be prescribed as local (creams, pessaries, rings) or systemic therapy (oral drugs, transdermal patches and gels, implants). Hormonal products available in such preparations may contain the following ingredients:
- Estrogen alone
- Combined estrogen and progestogen
- Selective estrogen receptor modulator (SERM)
- Tibolone, which contain estrogen, progestogen, and an androgen properties
- Combination of estrogen and SERM.

The estrogens most commonly prescribed are conjugated equine estrogen (CEE) that may be equine or synthetic, micronized 17β estradiol, and ethinyl estradiol. Natural progesterone that is micronized progesterone or dihydrogesterone have better safety profile than other progestines such as MPA and norethindrone acetate.

The various schedules of hormone therapy include the following:
- Estrogen alone taken daily
- *Cyclic or sequential regimens*: Progestogen is added for 10-14 days every 4 weeks with estrogen
- Continuous combined regimens: Estrogen and progestogen are taken daily.

Dose

"Standard" doses of estrogen given daily, such as 17-beta estradiol (oral 1 mg/day or transdermal 0.05 mg/day) are adequate for symptom relief in the majority of women.[6,13,14] An exception is younger women after bilateral oophorectomy. They often require higher doses (e.g., 2 mg oral estradiol or 0.1 mg transdermal estradiol or their equivalent) for the first 2-3 years after surgery; the dose can subsequently be tapered down. Oral CEE (0.625 mg/day) was commonly used in the past (and in WHI), but is prescribed less often now.

In the past, a "one-size-fits-all" approach to estrogen dosing in postmenopausal women was used, e.g., all women were started on the same dose ("standard doses"), and if symptoms were relieved, that dose was continued indefinitely. However, the current approach is to start with lower doses, such as transdermal estradiol (0.025 mg) or oral estradiol (0.5 mg/day), and titrate up to relieve symptoms. This approach does not apply to women with POI, which requires a higher daily dose.

Lower doses are associated with less vaginal bleeding, breast tenderness[15] fewer effects on coagulation and inflammatory markers, and a possible lower risk of stroke and VTE than standard-dose therapy.[16] The lowest available transdermal estradiol dose is 0.014 mg; it is approved for prevention of bone loss. However, approximately 50% of women derive some benefit for hot flashes.[17]

Progestins

All women with an intact uterus need a progestin to be added to their estrogen to prevent endometrial hyperplasia, which can occur after as little as 6 months of unopposed estrogen. Women who have undergone hysterectomy should not receive a progestin, as there are no other health benefits other than prevention of endometrial hyperplasia and carcinoma.

Dosing: The first choice of progestin is oral natural micronized progesterone [200 mg/day for 12 days/month (i.e., a cyclic regimen that is designed to mimic the normal luteal phase of premenopausal women) or 100 mg daily micronized (continuous regimen)]. Progesterone should be taken at bedtime as some of its metabolites are associated with somnolence. There are reasons to believe that natural progesterone is safer for the cardiovascular system (no adverse lipid effects) and possibly the breast. Women taking lower doses of estrogen (e.g., 0.014 mg transdermal estradiol) require very little progestin (a 12-day course every 6–12 months.[18] But this regimen is better to avoid as unscheduled bleeding might occur.

The most extensively studied formulation for endometrial protection is the synthetic progestin used in the WHI, MPA (MPA; 2.5 mg daily). While MPA is endometrial protective, it was associated with an excess risk of coronary heart disease (CHD) and breast cancer when administered with conjugated estrogen in the WHI. In addition, regimens using continuous versus cyclic MPA may be associated with a higher risk of breast cancer. Therefore, natural progesterone or dihydrogesterone are the choice of progesterone.

Vaginal progesterone inserts are sometimes tried, but endometrial safety data are limited.[19]

Estrogen

Estrogen can be used systemically as oral CEE, estradiol valerate, estrone sulfate or micronized estradiol; transdermal estradiol (patches, gels, spray); a vaginal estradiol ring; and as implanted estradiol pellets. Vaginal estrogen is used exclusively for the treatment of genitourinary syndrome of menopause or of urogenital atrophy. In Bangladesh, oral and transdermal route are popular.

Oral Estrogen Preparations

Advantages include:
- Very effective
- Convenience, and
- Reliable absorption for most users.

Disadvantages include:
- Slight increased of risk of VTE disease
- Slight increased risk of cholelithiasis
- Increased thyroid binding globulin (TBG)—may need to adjust thyroxine dose.

Transdermal Estradiol Preparations

Advantages include:
- Avoidance of gut and first-pass hepatic metabolism: No change in sex hormone-binding globulin (SHBG) or TBG, null effect on hepatic coagulation proteins
- Little/no increase in VTE disease
- Lower total dose
- Convenient for some women (e.g., once- or twice-a-week patch).

Disadvantages include:
- Patches may cause skin irritation and rarely general allergic reaction
- Gel can be "sticky" and inconvenient, occasionally poorly absorbed
- Women may forget to change twice-weekly patch.

Progestogen

Progestogen therapy is required for all women who have not had a hysterectomy. Progestogens include micronized progesterone and the synthetic progestins. There is evidence that supports micronized progesterone as being safer than synthetic progestin therapy in terms of breast cancer and cardiovascular disease risk.[20,21]

Micronized progesterone is taken either orally or the same capsule can be used as an intravaginal pessary. Synthetic progestins are mostly taken orally, separately or combined with oral estrogen, or in a combined estradiol-progestin patch.

The LNG-IUD is available in some countries also in Bangladesh and in appropriate circumstances is an excellent option for progestin effects to be achieved in the endometrium protection, with minimization of systemic side-effects.

Some,[22] but not all studies[23] indicate that, if a sufficient amount of trans-dermal progesterone can be administered, it may alleviate vasomotor symptoms and afford endometrial protection in the short term, but long-term benefit and safety need to be established. Also it is not available in Bangladesh.

■ MANAGING CLINICAL SIDE-EFFECTS OF MHT THERAPY

Common adverse effects of estrogen include nausea, headache, and breast tenderness. Combined estrogen–progestogen therapy sometimes can result in irregular bleeding.

Progestin therapy may cause lowered mood or irritability. When this occurs, either the dose needs to be reduced or the patient needs to be switched to another progestin. Micronized progesterone may result in less adverse mood effects.

Initiating treatment with low-dose estrogen will minimize the likelihood of adverse effects. Transdermal estrogen is less likely than oral estrogen to cause nausea. Changing from one estrogen regimen to another in many cases can alleviate certain adverse effects.

All women using systemic MHT require medical review every 6 months. Review should include updating medical history and a routine general health and breast check. Investigations should be individually assessed with at least annual mammography.

Bone densitometry measurement (DXA) should be performed where indicated.

All unexpected vaginal bleeding warrants investigation and, when appropriate, specialist referral. Transvaginal ultrasound and/or endometrial biopsy is required if there is any excessive or prolonged bleeding 3–6 months after commencing MHT.

The need for ongoing MHT, the formulation and dose requirement should be regularly reviewed.

Effectiveness

Estrogen therapy alleviates VMS and the other commonly reported symptoms of the menopause in 96% of women. Low-dose therapy can be highly effective.

Treatment Tips

If symptoms persist on high-dose oral therapy, there is no point increasing the dose if SHBG is high, as the administered estrogen will just be bound by the SHBG. Switch to nonoral.

If symptoms persist on high-dose, nonoral therapy, check serum estradiol to be sure the patient is actually absorbing the administered dose.

Although there is substantial controversy about whether menopause causes depression or major mood disturbance, many women report alleviation of anxiety and improved well-being with the use of estrogen therapy. There is also evidence for improved sleep quality.

Tibolone

Tibolone is a unique chemical compound that provides an alternative to estrogen-progestin therapy. Tibolone itself has very weak actions. It is metabolized in the gut and target tissues to metabolites that exhibit estrogenic, progestogenic and androgenic actions. Therefore, it alleviates VMS, has favorable mood effects, treats urogenital atrophy and does not activate the endometrium—and therefore, does not cause vaginal bleeding. Tibolone can also be converted to an active form which has weak androgen action. As a result, women may experience an improvement in sexual interest and responsiveness when they use tibolone.[24] It is uncommon for women using tibolone to experience breast tenderness, and tibolone does not increase mammographic density. Tibolone prevents bone loss and has been shown to reduce fractures in older women.[25]

Tibolone should not be prescribed with other hormone therapy and is contraindicated in women with breast cancer.[25]

Occasionally, women report fluid retention and mild weight gain with tibolone. Vaginal bleeding or spotting may occur in women just after commencing tibolone; So, tibolone should be start dater 1 year of completion of menopause. However, this is uncommon.

Tibolone 1.25 mg/day has been associated with a small increase in the risk of ischemic stroke in older women 26. For women aged 60-69 years, the risk of stroke was 2.8/1,000 person-years for tibolone and 1.0/1,000 person-years for placebo.

Estrogen + Selective Estrogen Receptor Modulator

The combination of a SERM with estrogen has been described as a tissue-selective estrogen complex (TSEC) therapy. The first of these is approved in the USA: the oral combination of CEE 0.45 mg/day with 20 mg of bazedoxifene (BZE). This therapy alleviates VMS, alleviates urogenital atrophy, preserves bone and does not stimulate the endometrium such that vaginal bleeding is minimal.[26] Mastalgia is uncommon with this therapy. The incidence of VTE with CEE/BZE needs further clarification. An increase in VTE has been reported in studies of BZE alone[27] but not in studies of combined CEE/BZE.[28] This preparation is not available in Bangladesh.

Oral Therapy for Urogenital Atrophy

Ospemifene is a SERM that has been approved in the USA for the treatment of vulvovaginal atrophy in postmenopausal women. The recommended dose is 60 mg/day. Ospemifene has an estrogen-like effect in the vagina (increases superficial cells and decreases parabasal cells and lowers vaginal pH). It results in a small, but statistically significant reduction in dyspareunia.[29] The most common adverse effect of ospemifene is VMS, which has been reported to occur in 10% of treated women.[30]

Potential risks of HT in postmenopausal women include the following:
- *Breast cancer*: Use of combined HT; study results inconsistent, but emerging consensus of slightly increased risk for breast cancer similar to that associated with natural late menopause—comes into effect after at least 5 years of continuous HT.[31]
- *Endometrial cancer[32] and uterine hyperplasia and cancer*: Use of HT based on unopposed estrogen.

- *Thromboembolism*: Use of combined or estrogen-only HT.
- *Biliary pathology*: Use of estrogen only or combined estrogen/progestogen HT.[33]

How to Monitor a Woman Who is on MHT?

Menopause practitioners often report that bringing patients back within a few months after initiating MHT may be useful to assess symptom response and tolerance, allowing for dose adjustment if needed. Thereafter, annual reassessment of the balance of benefits and risks individualized to each woman's particular health circumstances is generally advised. Annual reassessment typically includes a clinical breast examination, mammogram (for women 40 years and older), pelvic examination (if indicated), symptom assessment, review of intervening health concerns, family medical history, discussion of any new research findings, and reassessment of the woman's preferences.

NONHORMONAL OPTIONS WITH EVIDENCE TO SUPPORT EFFICACY

Many women are interested to take nonhormonal preparation than hormonal preparation. An array of nonhormonal therapies is recommended for the treatment of VMS, few of which have evidence to support efficacy.

Selective Serotonin Reuptake Inhibitors and Serotonin-Norepinephrine Reuptake Inhibitors

Selective serotonin reuptake inhibitors (SSRIs) and serotonin-norepinephrine reuptake inhibitors (SNRIs) are effective in some, but not all women with VMS, and have the added benefit of improving mood and well-being. Recommended doses are listed in the Toolkit.

A recent systematic review and meta-analysis concluded: "SSRI use is associated with modest improvement in the severity and frequency of hot flushes but can also be associated with the typical profile of SSRI adverse effects."[34]

Clonidine

Clonidine is sometimes prescribed for the management of VMS for women who cannot take estrogen. Studies of clonidine for VMS have been small and most show no benefit over placebo.[35] A dose of 100–150 μg/day may be effective in some women, although the effect is modes.[36] The most common side-effect, dry mouth, is dose-related.

Gabapentin

Gabapentin is an antiepileptic that also is indicated for the treatment of neuropathic pain. It has been found in several studies to reduce VMS in postmenopausal women in doses of 300–900 mg/day.[37] The anxiolytic effects of gabapentin may also be beneficial for some women. Side-effects include headache, dizziness and somnolence and are dose-related. Preliminary data also support the off-label use of *pregabalin*, in a dose of 75–150 mg twice daily, for the treatment of VMS.[38]

Hypnosis

Hypnosis has been shown to diminish VMS in a study of postmenopausal women.[39] Although this needs further verification, it can be considered as a treatment option for women who are unable to take hormone therapy and who have not achieved a satisfactory outcome with other nonhormonal interventions.

Cognitive Behavior Therapy

Cognitive behavior therapy (CBT) employs psychotherapeutic behavior modification to help women deal with VMS. In expert hands, CBT has been shown to significantly reduce VMS.[40]

Stellate Ganglion Blockade

Blockade of the stellate ganglion at the anterolateral aspect of the C6 vertebra on the right side under fluoroscopy has been shown to alleviate severe VMS for up to 12 weeks.[41] This option could be considered for women with severe, debilitating VMS when other treatments are contraindicated or ineffective and where expertise in this procedure is available.

■ ANDROGEN THERAPY

Testosterone

There is no level of testosterone below which a woman can be said to be androgen-deficient, and a "testosterone deficiency syndrome" has never been biochemically defined. However, several randomized, clinical trials have demonstrated efficacy of testosterone, in doses appropriate for women, for the treatment of low sexual desire/arousal disorder. This has been shown for naturally and surgically menopausal women, and for MHT users and nonusers.[42]

Although a transdermal patch, releasing 300 ou of testosterone per day, was approved for surgically menopausal women. Testosterone pellets are no longer available. A transdermal testosterone cream (AndroFeme 1%) is available in Australia, although it has not been approved by the Australian Therapeutics Goods Administration. The recommended starting dose is 0.5 mL/day, applied to the lower torso/upper thigh. It is essential that testosterone levels are monitored shortly after commencement of treatment and regularly during treatment (6-monthly) as absorption is variable. Blood levels of calculated free testosterone should be kept below the upper limit of the range for premenopausal women.

Women should be advised that when testosterone is administered in a dose that results in levels within the normal female range, the effects of treatment usually do not emerge for 6–8 weeks. Therefore treatment needs to be continued at least this long as a therapeutic trial. If no benefit is seen by 6 months, treatment should be discontinued.

Side effects of testosterone therapy are rare when treatment is prescribed for appropriately selected women and given in the appropriate dose. Side effects from *excessive* dosage can include masculinization with acne and excess body hair, fluid retention, and cliteromegaly. These side effects are rare if the appropriate dose of testosterone is administered.

Women with severe acne or severe excess body hair should not use testosterone. Similarly, women who are pregnant, lactating or who have a suspected cancer should not use testosterone as a standard precaution.

Dehydroepiandrosterone

Dehydroepiandrosterone was popularized in the 1990s as a treatment to improve well-being, sexual function, and possibly reduce menopausal symptoms. Subsequent randomized, placebo-controlled trials have not shown oral DHEA to be effective as a treatment for estrogen deficiency symptoms in postmenopausal women. It has been shown to be no more effective than placebo for low sexual desire, diminished well-being, and cognitive function.[43] Data to support the routine prescription of DHEA to postmenopausal women with adrenal insufficiency are also lacking.[44]

There is no high-quality, consistent evidence that yoga, paced respiration, acupuncture, exercise, stress reduction, relaxation therapy, and alternative therapies such as black cohosh, botanical products, omega-3 fatty acid supplements, and dietary Chinese herbs benefit patients more than placebo.

■ KEY MESSAGES

The science of MHT is evolving, and it is important to stay informed and keep an open perspective of understanding about MHT. Important factors to take into consideration include the woman's age, type and timing of menopause, impact of symptoms on quality-of-life, family history/medical history, and personal preferences:

- MHT can then be recommended to women who are at the right age, have no contraindications, and have low cardiovascular and breast cancer risks.
- MHT safely can be used for duration 5 years. However, extended use is sometimes necessary for women with persistent, severe hot flashes there is no hard and fast rule that MHT can not be used for more than 5 years.

- Women with POI should continue MHT until the average of menopause, e.g., age 51 years, to decrease the risk of premature CVD, stroke, osteoporosis, and dementia.
- However, there are strong data to suggest that use of estrogen within the first 10 years of clinical menopause may reduce the risks of CVD and all type mortality, osteoporosis, and other chronic illness.
- All types and routes of estrogen are equally effective for hot flashes. 17-beta estradiol is preferable over CEEs, because it is structurally identical (bioidentical) to the main estrogen secreted by the ovary.
- The transdermal route is particularly important in women with hypertriglyceridemia, active gallbladder disease, without a personal history of VTE. The baseline risk of both VTE and stroke is very low in otherwise healthy, young postmenopausal women.
- Oral estradiol in healthy woman is a safe and reasonable option for patients who prefer an oral preparation over a transdermal one (cost or personal preference).
- For women with an intact uterus who are starting MHT and therefore, require a progestin, micronized progesterone should be chosen as first-line progestin. It is effective to prevent endometrial hyperplasia, it is metabolically neutral, and does not appear to increase the risk of either breast cancer or CHD.
- For women who experience recurrent, bothersome hot flashes after stopping estrogen, initially she may try nonhormonal options. However, if this approach is unsuccessful and symptoms persist, she may resume MHT at the lowest dose possible in carefully selected women.
- Counseling with risks and benefits of MHT needs to be discussed so that women could be empowered to have informed choice of MHT.

REFERENCES

1. Manson JE, Chlebowski RT, Stefanick ML, Aragaki AK, Rossouw JE, Prentice RL, et al. Menopausal hormone therapy and health outcomes during the intervention and extended poststopping phases of the Women's Health Initiative randomized trials. JAMA. 2013;310(13):1353-68.
2. Mikkola TS, Clarkson TB. Estrogen replacement therapy, atherosclerosis, and vascular function. Cardiovasc Res. 2002;53(3):605-19.
3. ACOG committee opinion no. 565. Hormone therapy and heart disease. Obstet Gynecol. 2013;121(6):1407-10.
4. The American Academy of Family Physicians. Hormone replacement therapy. [online] Available from: https://www.aafp.org/patient-care/clinical-recommendations/all/hrt.html [Last accessed March, 2021].
5. Hodis HN, Collins P, Mack WJ, Schierbeck LL. The window of opportunity for coronary heart disease prevention with hormone therapy: past, present and future in perspective. Climacteric. 2012;15:217-28.
6. Nelson HD. Commonly used types of postmenopausal estrogen for treatment of hot flashes: scientific review. JAMA. 2004;291:1610.
7. National Cancer institute. Breast Cancer Risk Assessment tool. [online] Available from: https://www.cancer.gov/bcrisktool [Last accessed March, 2021].

8. Gass MLS, Stuenkel CA, Utian WH, LaCroix A, Liu JH, Shifren JL, et al. Use of compounded hormone therapy in the United States: report of The North American Menopause Society Survey. Menopause. 2015;22:1276-85.
9. Stuenkel CA, Davis SR, Gompel A, Lumsden MA, Murad MH, Pinkerton JAV, et al. Treatment of symptoms of the menopause: an endocrine society clinical practice guideline. J Clin Endocrinol Metab. 2015;100:3975-4011.
10. Gompel A. Micronized progesterone and its impact on the endometrium and breast vs. progestogens. Climacteric. 2012;15:18-25.
11. Baber R, Panay N, Fenton A, IMS Writing Grp, IMS Writing Group. 2016 IMS recommendations on women's midlife health and menopause hormone therapy. Climacteric. 2016;19:109-50.
12. de Villiers TJ, Gass ML, Haines CJ, Hall JE, Lobo RA, Pierroz DD, et al. Global Consensus Statement on menopausal hormone therapy. Climacteric. 2013;16:203-4.
13. Steingold KA, Laufer L, Chetkowski RJ, DeFazio JD, Matt DW, Meldrum DR, et al. Treatment of hot flashes with transdermal estradiol administration. J Clin Endocrinol Metab. 1985;61:627.
14. Maclennan AH, Broadbent JL, Lester S, Moore V. Oral oestrogen and combined oestrogen/progestogen therapy versus placebo for hot flushes. Cochrane Database Syst Rev. 2004;CD002978.
15. Ettinger B. Vasomotor symptom relief versus unwanted effects: role of estrogen dosage. Am J Med. 2005;118 (Suppl 12B):74.
16. Grodstein F, Manson JE, Stampfer MJ, Rexrode K. Postmenopausal hormone therapy and stroke: role of time since menopause and age at initiation of hormone therapy. Arch Intern Med. 2008;168:861.
17. Bachmann GA, Schaefers M, Uddin A, Utian WH. Lowest effective transdermal 17beta-estradiol dose for relief of hot flushes in postmenopausal women: a randomized controlled trial. Obstet Gynecol. 2007;110:771.
18. Johnson SR, Ettinger B, Macer JL, Ensrud KE, Quan J, Grady D. Uterine and vaginal effects of unopposed ultralow-dose transdermal estradiol. Obstet Gynecol. 2005;105:779.
19. Stanczyk FZ, Hapgood JP, Winer S, Mishell DR Jr. Progestogens used in postmenopausal hormone therapy: differences in their pharmacological properties, intracellular actions, and clinical effects. Endocr Rev. 2013;34(2):171-208.
20. Simon JA. What if the Women's Health Initiative had used transdermal estradiol and oral progesterone instead? Menopause. 2014;21:769-83.
21. Fournier A, Fabre A, Mesrine S, Boutron-Ruault MC, Berrino F, Clavel-Chapelon F. Use of different postmenopausal hormone therapies and risk of histology- and hormone receptor-defined invasive breast cancer. J Clin Oncol. 2008;26:1260-8.
22. Leonetti HB, Wilson KJ, Anasti JN. Topical progesterone cream has an antiproliferative effect on estrogen stimulated endometrium. Fertil Steril. 2003;79:221-2.
23. Cooper A, Spencer MI, Whitehead M, Ross D, Barnard GJR, Collins WP. Systemic absorption of progesterone from Progest cream in postmenopausal women. Lancet. 1998;351:125.
24. Nijland EA, Weijmar Schultz WC, Nathorst-Boos J, Helmond FA, Van Lunsen RH, Palacios S, et al. Tibolone and transdermal E2/NETA for the treatment of female sexual dysfunction in naturally menopausal women: results of a randomized active-controlled trial. J Sex Med. 2008;5:646-56.
25. Cummings SR, Ettinger B, Delmas PD, Kenemans P, Stathopoulos V, Verweij P, et al. The effects of tibolone in older postmenopausal women. N Engl J Med. 2008;359:697-708.
26. Mirkin S, Komm BS, Pan K, Chines AA. Effects of bazedoxifene/conjugated estrogens on endometrial safety and bone in postmenopausal women. Climacteric. 2013;16:338-46.

27. de Villiers TJ, Chines AA, Palacios S, Lips P, Sawicki AZ, Levine AB, et al. Safety and tolerability of bazedoxifene in postmenopausal women with osteoporosis: results of a 5-year, randomized, placebo-controlled phase 3 trial. Osteoporos Int. 2011;22:567-76.
28. Pinkerton JV, Komm BS, Mirkin S. Tissue selective estrogen complex combinations with bazedoxifene/conjugated estrogens as a model. Climacteric. 2013;16:618-28.
29. Portman DJ, Bachmann GA, Simon JA. Ospemifene, a novel selective estrogen receptor modulator for treating dyspareunia associated with postmenopausal vulvar and vaginal atrophy. Menopause. 2013;20:623-30.
30. Simon J, Portman D, Mabey RG Jr. Long-term safety of ospemifene (52-week extension) in the treatment of vulvar and vaginal atrophy in hysterectomized postmenopausal women. Maturitas. 2014;77:274-81.
31. La Vecchia C, Brinton LA, McTiernan A. Cancer risk in menopausal women. Best Pract Res Clin Obstet Gynaecol. 2002;16(3):293-307.
32. Ziel HK, Finkle WD. Increased risk of endometrial carcinoma among users of conjugated estrogens. N Engl J Med. 1975;293(23):1167-70.
33. Cirillo DJ, Wallace RB, Rodabough RJ, Greenland P, LaCroix AZ, Limacher MC, et al. Effect of estrogen therapy on gallbladder disease. JAMA. 2005;293(3):330-9.
34. Shams T, Firwana B, Habib F, Alshahrani A, Alnouh B, Murad MH, et al. SSRIs for hot flashes: a systematic review and meta-analysis of randomized trials. J Gen Intern Med. 2014;29:204-13.
35. Lindsay R, Hart DM. Failure of response of menopausal vasomotor symptoms to clonidine. Maturitas. 1978;1:21-5.
36. Pandya KJ, Raubertas RF, Flynn PJ, Hynes HE, Rosenbluth RJ, Kirshner JJ, et al. Oral clonidine in postmenopausal patients with breast cancer experiencing tamoxifen-induced hot flashes: a University of Rochester Cancer Center Community Clinical Oncology Program study. Ann Intern Med. 2000;132:788-93.
37. Pandya KJ, Morrow GR, Roscoe JA, Zhao H, Hickok JT, Pajon E, et al. Gabapentin for hot flashes in 420 women with breast cancer: a randomised double-blind placebo-controlled trial. Lancet. 2005;366:818-24.
38. Nguyen ML. The use of pregabalin in the treatment of hot flashes. Can Pharm J. 2013;146:193-6.
39. Elkins GR, Fisher WI, Johnson AK, Carpenter JS, Keith TZ. Clinical hypnosis in the treatment of postmenopausal hot flashes: a randomized controlled trial. Menopause. 2013;20:291-8.
40. Ayers B, Hunter MS. Health-related quality of life of women with menopausal hot flushes and night sweats. Climacteric. 2013;16:235-9.
41. Lipov EG, Joshi JR, Sanders S, Wilcox K, Lipov S, Xie H, et al. Effects of stellate-ganglion block on hot flushes and night awakenings in survivors of breast cancer: a pilot study. Lancet Oncol. 2008;9:523-32.
42. Panay N, Al-Azzawi F, Bouchard C, Davis SR, Eden J, Lodhi I, et al. Testosterone treatment of HSDD in naturally menopausal women: the ADORE study. Climacteric. 2010;13:121-31.
43. Davis SR, Panjari M, Stanczyk FZ. DHEA replacement for postmenopausal women. J Clin Endocrinol Metab. 2011;96:1642-53.
44. Alkatib AA, Cosma M, Elamin MB, Erickson D, Swiglo BA, Erwin PJ, et al. A systematic review and meta-analysis of randomized placebo-controlled trials of DHEA treatment effects on quality of life in women with adrenal insufficiency. J Clin Endocrinol Metab. 2009;94:3676-81.

Index

Page numbers followed by *f* refer to figure, and *t* refer to table.

A

Abaloparatide 73
Acanthosis nigricans 159
Acetylcholinesterase inhibitor 100
Acne, types of 122
Acupuncture 38
Adiposity, abdominal 21
Adrenal insufficiency 142
Agnosia 95
Alcohol 98
Alendronate 74
Alopecia 123
Alzheimer's disease 8, 95
Amentia 95
American Academy of Family Physicians 190
American Academy of Neurology 96
American Association of Sexuality Educators, Counselors, and Therapists 55
American College of Cardiology 193
American College of Obstetricians and Gynecologists 115, 172
American Heart Association 22, 159, 193
American Society for Reproductive Medicine 115
Anabolic agents 74
Anagen hair 120
Androgen 10
  therapy 203
Androgenetic alopecia 124
Androstenedione 9
Angelica sinensis 38
Angina, types of 7
Angiotensin
  converting enzyme inhibitors 163
  receptor blockers 163
Anovulation, chronic 169
Antiaging cream 122
Anticoagulant therapy 171
Antidepressant 56, 100
Antihypertensive 164
Anti-müllerian hormone 9, 11, 141
Antiplatelets 164
Antiresorptive drugs 73
Antral follicle count 141
Anxiety 92, 134, 135
Aphasia 95
Apraxia 95
ASCOT technique 151
Atheroma 82*f*
Atherosclerotic cardiovascular disease 156
Atrophic vaginitis 175
Atrophic vulvovaginitis 125
Atrophy 169
Atypia 174, 176

B

Back pain 65
Bacterial vaginosis 108
Barrier method 111, 113
Bazedoxifene 35, 201
Biliary pathology 202
Bi-manual vaginal examination 173
Biopsy, endometrial 172
Biopsychosocial model 103
Bisphosphonates, contraindications of 74
Bladder 171
Bleeding disorder 169
Bloating 131
Blood
  chemistry 67
  pressure 33, 157, 159, 191
    control 163
    diastolic 159
    systolic 87, 159
  sugar
    fasting 157
    profile 192
Body
  fat distribution 164
  mass index 23, 191
  pain 65
Bodyache 21

Bone
  densitometry measurement 200
  health 61
  loss 63f, 193
    prevention of 148
  matrix 63
  mineral density 62, 69, 115, 144
  mineral density around menopause, rate of 64f
  pain 65
  turnover markers 68, 69
Brain 92
  fog 92, 131
Breast
  cancer 21, 35, 112, 113, 180, 182, 183, 193, 201
    history of 193
    invasive 181
    risk, evaluate of 193
    survivors 37
  examination 191
  pain 1
Breath, shortness of 159
Brittle nail syndrome 125
Broad-spectrum sunscreen 122
Bupropion 107
Burning sensation 125

C

Calcitriol 74
Calcium 24, 62
  absorption of 25
  recommendation of 71t
  use, practical aspect of 71
Cancer 169, 171, 201
  endometrial 168, 169, 172, 181, 186, 193, 201
Carcinoma 184
  endometrial 176
  hereditary nonpolyposis colorectal 169
Cardiovascular disease 7, 9, 15, 81, 144, 156, 180, 190, 193
  development of 7
  prevention of 26, 87, 150
  screen 87
Cardiovascular fitness 28
Cardiovascular health 81
Cardiovascular risk 193
Celiac disease 142

Centers for Disease Control and Prevention 110
Ceramides 122
Cervical
  cancer 123, 168
  carcinoma 176
  cytology 174
  polyp 168
  ulcer 168
Chemotherapy 11
Chest pain 159
Cholesterol 81
Clonidine 37, 151, 202
Cognitive behavioral therapy 37, 137, 203
Cognitive disorders 2
Colon cancer 180
Colorectal cancer 181, 185
Combined estrogen-progestin therapy 181
  lower doses of 184
Combined oral contraceptives 110, 111, 149
Communicable diseases, death patterns of 84f
Complete blood count 192
Comprehensive metabolic panel 143
Computed tomography 174
  quantitative 69
Conjugated estrogen 35
Contraception 149
  benefits of 114
Contraceptive
  implant 113
  options of 110
Copper intrauterine device 113
Coronary heart disease 35, 81, 144, 180, 198
  prevention of 25
  symptoms of 7
Cowden syndrome 169
C-reactive protein 160
Creatinine 143
Cytomegalovirus 142

D

Danish Osteoporosis Prevention Study 182
Dehydroepiandrosterone 11, 44, 103, 148, 204
  sulfate 31

Dementia 93, 94, 180
Denosumab 74
Dental checkup 191
Depot-medroxyprogesterone acetate 110, 113
Depression 1, 31, 92, 134, 135, 137
Depressive disorders, symptoms of 137
Diabetes mellitus 17, 21, 156, 159, 163, 169
Diet 162, 163
Digital rectal examination 173
Dioscorea villosa 38
Disturbed sleep 92
Dizziness 36
Docosahexaenoic acid 161
Drospirenone 111
Dry eye disease 185
Dry skin 121
Dual-energy X-ray absorptiometry 143
Dyslipidemia 163
   severe 159
Dysmenorrhea 114
Dyspareunia 6, 14, 52, 104, 125

E

Edema 191
Eicosapentaenoic acid 161
Electrocardiogram 144
Electrocardiography 192
Electrolytes 143
Emergency contraception 114
Endogenous estrogen, levels of 83
Endometrial intraepithelial neoplasia 171
Endometrial protection 196
Endometrial safety 176
Endometrial thickness 170, 175
Equine estrogen 51
Estradiol 182
Estrogen 31, 92, 110, 119, 181, 197, 198, 201
   deficiency 47*f*
   effect of 46
   loss of 103, 108
   only therapy 169
   protects 93
   secreting tumor 169
   therapy 50, 165, 185
Exercise 25, 38, 71, 88
Eyes 8, 185
   checkup 191

F

Facial hair 121
Fallopian tube 171
Fasting high-density lipoprotein cholesterol 157
Fat distribution, changes of 84*f*
Fatigue 36
Female genitourinary system, anatomy of 45*f*
Female sexual
   dysfunction 103
   interest 103
   orgasmic disorder 103
Female sexuality, role on 103
Fertility issues 150
Follicle-stimulating hormone 11, 16, 31, 92, 140
Fractures 180
   osteoporosis related 75
Fragile X syndrome 142
Free fatty acids 158
Frontal fibrosing alopecia 126

G

Gabapentin 56, 151, 202
Galactosemia 142
Genital itching 123
Genito-pelvic pain 103
Genitourinary atrophy symptoms 19
Genitourinary dysfunction 2
Genitourinary symptoms 6, 57
Glucose, fasting 159
Glycosaminoglycans, polymerization of 119

H

Hair
   loss, female pattern 124
   thinning of 121
Hashimoto's thyroiditis, autoimmune 142
Heart
   auscultation of 191
   diseases 86
   health 33
   normal 82*f*
Height 191
Hemography 192
Hemorrhoids 171

High-density lipoprotein 7
   cholesterol 159
Hip fracture 181
   risk of 70
Hirsutism 159
Hormonal concentrations 32
Hormonal tests 16
Hormone
   deficiency, effect of 131
   estrogen 103
   measurement of 16, 17
   replacement therapy 76, 93, 119, 129, 137, 141, 190
   therapy 72, 115, 165
      postmenopausal 171
      principles of 145
Hot flashes 123
Human chorionic gonadotropin 19
Human immunodeficiency virus 142
Human monoclonal immunoglobulin G 77
Hyperglycemia 159
Hyperhidrosis 123
Hyperplasia 174, 176
   endometrial 168, 170, 171, 184
Hypertension 159, 163, 169
   treatment of 161
Hypertriglyceridemia 159
Hypnosis 203
Hypoactive sexual desire disorder 144
Hypocalcemia 74
Hysterectomy 174, 175
Hysteroscopy 170, 173

I

Ibandronate 74
Impaired glucose tolerance 156
Impaired orgasm 104
In vitro fertilization 151
Infection 168, 171
Inflammation 123
Inflammatory bowel disease 142, 171
Insomnia 1, 5, 135
   chronic 136
International Diabetes Foundation 158
International Menopause Society 147, 180
Intraepithelial neoplasia 171
Intrauterine contraceptive devices 14, 111
Intravaginal prasterone 53

Iron deficiency 17
Irregular menses 1, 4
Irreversible tissue atrophy 45
Irritation 125
Itching 125
   during menopause, types of 123

J

Joints 7
   pains 131

K

Keratoderma climacteric 125
Kinmen Women-Health Investigation 93
Kronos Early Estrogen Prevention Study 182

L

Labial fusion 125
Laser
   administration, technique of 56f
   newer generation of 54
   therapy 54
Lean protein 27
Leiomyomata uteri 171
Levonorgestrel 112
   releasing intrauterine system 35, 112, 174, 184, 195
Lipid-lowering agents 164
Liver
   disease, active 193
   function test 143
Long-acting reversible contraception methods 114
Low-density lipoprotein 81, 146
   cholesterol 160
Lower sex drive 108
Lubricants 50
Lung, auscultation of 191
Luteinizing hormone 11
   receptor 140
Lynch syndrome 169

M

Magnesium 24, 62
Magnetic resonance imaging 174
Malaria 142
Mammography 192, 193

Medical menopause 18
Mediterranean diet 97
Medroxyprogesterone 184
  acetate 86
Memory
  loss 8, 97
  problems 92, 95
Menarche, early 169
Menopausal flushing 125
Menopausal hormone therapy 54, 81, 89, 99, 115, 141, 176, 180, 186, 190, 195, 197
  benefits of 180
  formulations 197
  risk of 180
Menopausal hormone treatment 85
  role of 85
Menopausal symptoms 9, 16, 17, 30, 49, 127
Menopausal transition 3, 14, 18, 99
Menopause 1, 10, 11, 30, 44, 61, 68, 81, 83, 92, 96, 103, 104, 119, 131, 156
  consequences of 4
  diagnosis of 14, 18
  effects of 83*f*
  endocrine changes after 11*t*
  genitourinary syndrome of 6, 44, 46, 55, 61, 144, 148
  hormone therapy 6, 33, 34, 108, 134
    indiscriminate use of 168
  impact of 83
  late 169
  management of 116
  natural 10, 18
  physiological changes of 9, 121, 122
  physiology of 8
  premature 9
  primary skin disorders of 123
  progression of 92
  status 64
  symptoms 15
    duration of 32
  transition 10
Menorrhagia 113, 114
Menstrual cycle 22
Menstrual irregularities 4
Menstrual period 22
Mental
  activation 98
  depression, severe 103
  health 33, 131

Metabolic syndrome 7, 156, 157, 159, 165
  components of 156
  symptoms of 18
Metronidazole 122
Mind–body-based therapies 38
Mindfulness training 38
Moisturizers 50
Mood
  changes 1, 21
  disorders 5
Multiple hamartoma syndrome 169
Multiple sclerosis 142
Muscle
  mass 191
  strengthening activities 89
Myasthenia gravis 142
Myocardial infarction 112, 193
Myometrium abnormalities 173

N

National Cholesterol Education Program 156, 159
National Heart, Lung, and Blood Institute 159
National Institute for Health and Care Excellence 131
Nausea 36
Night sweats 21, 123
Nitric oxide 83, 146
Noncommunicable diseases, death patterns of 84*f*
Nonhormonal therapy 55*t*, 56
Nonobstructive coronary heart disease 7
North American Menopause Society 22, 115
Nutrients, essential 24
Nutrition 21, 97, 163

O

Obesity 7, 31, 158, 164, 169, 173
  abdominal 159
Oral bisphosphonate 74
Oral contraceptive pill 112, 149
Oral dehydroepiandrosterone 196
Oral emergency contraception 114
Oral estrogen preparations 198
Oral micronized progesterone 184

Ospemifene 53
Osteoporosis 6, 26, 61, 66, 81, 148, 180, 185
    causes of 67
    diagnosis of 65
    drugs for 73
    epidemiology of 61
    lifestyle modification 70
    preventive 70
    risk factors for 65
    treatment of 70, 74t
Osteoporotic disability, incidence of 62
Ovarian cancer 169, 171, 183
Ovarian estrogen production 1
Ovarian failure 119
Ovarian follicles, loss of 9
Ovarian function
    loss of 140
    permanent cessation of 1
Ovarian insufficiency 186
Ovarian rejuvenation 151
Ovarian rescue 151
Ovarian theca cell, postmenopausal 9
Ovaries 140
Oxybutynin 37, 151

P

Painful intercourse 125
Painful urination 125
Papanicolaou test 192
Parathyroid hormone 73, 143
Paroxetine 151
Pelvic
    examination 191
    floor, impact of menopause on 47f
    inflammatory diseases 113
    physical therapy 56
    radiation 11
Penetration disorder 103
Perimenopause 10, 14, 18
Peripheral neuropathy 159
Pharmacotherapy 99
Phosphate 62
Phytoestrogens 169
Pimples 122
Pioglitazone 164
Plasma-rich protein 57
Pneumonia 61

Polycyclic aromatic hydrocarbon exposure 142
Polypectomy, hysteroscopic 170
Polyps 170
    endometrial 168, 175
Posterior fourchette, recurrent fissures of 125
Postmenopausal bleeding 52, 168
    differential diagnosis of 168
Postmenopause 3, 10
Postnatal depression 134
Postradiation therapy 171
Prasterone cream 52
Premature ovarian
    failure 140, 147f, 186
    insufficiency 95, 140, 141, 142, 143, 145, 150, 152
    diagnosis of 142
Premenstrual dysphoric disorder 134
Premenstrual syndrome 134
Primary ovarian insufficiency 11, 140, 190
Primary sleep disorders 135
Progesterone 35, 92, 110, 146, 194
    medroxyprogesterone acetate 190
    natural 86
Progestins 198
    protective effect of 184
    therapy 200
Progestogen 146, 197, 199
    pill 110-112
Protein-derived energy 23
Pruritus 123, 129
Psychotherapy 99
Pulmonary embolism 112, 181, 193
Pulse 191

R

Raloxifene 74, 121
Randomized controlled trial 147
Rejuvenate orgasm system 57
Reproductive ageing workshop, stages of 4t
Reproductive life, end of 81
Resistant ovary syndrome 141
Restless legs syndrome 135
Retinoids cream 122
Retinopathy 159
Rheumatoid arthritis 142
Risedronate 74
Rosiglitazone 164

S

Saline infusion sonography 170, 174
Sarcopenia 8
Sclerostin inhibitors 73
Selective estrogen receptor modulator 53, 100, 121, 197, 201
Selective norepinephrine reuptake inhibitors 36
Selective serotonin reuptake inhibitors 137, 202
Senile alopecia 124
Serotonin reuptake inhibitors 56
Serotonin-norepinephrine reuptake inhibitors 202
Serum thyroid profile 192
Sex hormone-binding globulin 9, 11, 146
Sex therapy 55
Sexual and reproductive healthcare, faculty of 18, 113
Sexual behavior 104
Sexual dysfunction 14, 92
Sjögren's syndrome 142
Skin
    cancer 121
    care 119
    changes 7
        during menopause, pathophysiology of 119
    disorders, treatment of 127
Sleep 134
    disturbance 33, 135
    health 164
Smoking 32, 98
Sonogram 192
Speculum examination 173
Spine 191
Statins 164
Stellate ganglion blockade 39, 203
Stem cell therapies 151
Sterilization 113
    female 113
Straw system 4*t*
Stroke 144, 181, 182, 193
Sun-damaged skin, signs of 121
Superficial cells, loss of 46
Surgical menopause 18
Swelling 36
Systemic hormone replacement therapy 51
Systemic non-hormonal therapy 106

T

Tamoxifen 100, 168
    use 169
Teeth 8
Telogen effluvium 126
Teriparatide 73, 74
Testosterone 103, 107, 203
    cream 52
    loss of 103
    therapy 107
Thermoregulatory 31
Thromboembolic diseases 61
Thromboembolism 111, 202
Thyroid
    binding globulin 199
    disease 17
    stimulating hormone 143, 160
Tibolone 37, 106, 200
Tissue selective estrogen complexes 35
    therapy 201
Toxins, reduction of 98
Transdermal estradiol preparations 199
Transvaginal ultrasound 170, 173
Trichotillomania 127
Triglycerides 87, 157, 159, 160
T-score 66
    dual-energy X-ray absorptiometry 66*t*
Tubal ligations 111
Tuberculosis 142
Turner syndrome 142

U

Ulipristal acetate 114
Ultrasonography 192
    quantitative 69
Unwanted hair 122
Urea, serum 143
Urethra, diseases of 171
Urethritis 171
Urinalysis 192
Urinary tract infection 171
Urine and stool routine test 192
Urogenital atrophy, oral therapy for 201
Uterine
    bleeding, abnormal 113
    fibroids 113

hyperplasia 201
position 173
prolapse 168
sarcoma 168
Uterus, sarcomas of 171

V

Vagina, changes of 48, 49f
Vaginal atrophy 48, 168
Vaginal bleeding 193
Vaginal cancer 123, 169
Vaginal dehydroepiandrosterone 52
Vaginal dryness 50, 131
　symptoms of 14
Vaginal estrogen creams 108
Vaginal health 48
Vaginal mucosa
　changes of 47f
　histopathological changes of 51f
　improvement of 56f
Vaginal ring 110
Vaginal symptoms 131
Vaginal tears 125
Varicella 142
Varicose vein 191
Vasomotor symptoms 4, 15, 30, 33, 61
　risk factors for 31
Venlafaxine 151
Venous thromboembolism 35, 111, 146, 182, 193
Verbal memory 92
Vitamin
　A 25
　C 25
　D 24, 25, 56, 70, 71, 76
　　deficiency 75
　　practical points of 71
　E 24
　K 24
Vulva, changes of 48
Vulvar cancer 123, 169
Vulvar lichen sclerosis 125
Vulvovaginal atrophy 21, 44, 106, 144
Vulvovaginal candidiasis 125

W

Waist circumference 157, 160, 191
Weight 191
　gain 1, 36
White skin 125
World Health Organization 21
Wound healing, impaired 124
Wrinkled skin 125

X

Xanthelasmas 159
Xanthomas 159

Y

Yoga 39

Z

Zinc 24
Zoledronic acid 74

EU GSPR Authorised Reprsentative
Logos Europe, 9 rue Nicolas Poussin
1700, La Rochelle, France
Phone: +33 (0) 6 67 93 73 78
E-mail: contact@logoseurope.eu

www.ingramcontent.com/pod-product-compliance
Ingram Content Group UK Ltd.
Pitfield, Milton Keynes, MK11 3LW, UK
UKHW050428150426
5217IPUK00019B/1290